Praise for *The Contagion Next Time*

"*The Contagion Next Time* offers a prescription for our health and well-being that is nothing less than the 'revolution of values' that Rev. Dr. Martin Luther King, Jr. called for in 1967. Sandro Galea's diagnosis rightly indicates that we must address poverty, inequality, and systemic racism to ensure good health. Deeply engaging and insightful, this book is required reading to ensure that we not only survive the next pandemic, but thrive for generations to come."
— **Shailly Gupta Barnes**, Policy Director, Kairos Center and the Poor People's Campaign

"Sandro Galea's compelling and compassionate new book shows us how we must create a strong foundation in order to avert further pandemics. He urges us to address our pervasive but neglected nonmedical issues, including the American tradition of proud individualism that prevents us from recognizing how our health is interconnected, and reminds us, vividly, that until we begin to invest in our communal physical and mental health, we will remain vulnerable to future threats."
— **Rosalynn Carter**, former First Lady

"Sandro Galea's book proves it is possible for us to build a healthier world after Covid-19—and the first step is to protect the most vulnerable, whether they're in our own neighborhoods or across the globe. *The Contagion Next Time* is truly a must read."
— **Katie Couric**, award-winning journalist

"*The Contagion Next Time* brings into focus why we have never been able to realize an equitable response during pandemics and what change agents can do to create more healthy, equitable, and empowered communities. Sandro Galea's illuminating and pathbreaking work will shape the global conversation around the forces that shape health for generations to come."
— **Daniel E. Dawes**, Executive Director, Satcher Health Leadership Institute at Morehouse School of Medicine and author of *The Political Determinants of Health*

THE CONTAGION
NEXT TIME

THE
CONTAGION
NEXT TIME

SANDRO GALEA

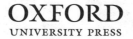

OXFORD
UNIVERSITY PRESS

Oxford University Press is a department of the University of Oxford. It furthers the University's objective of excellence in research, scholarship, and education by publishing worldwide. Oxford is a registered trade mark of Oxford University Press in the UK and certain other countries.

Published in the United States of America by Oxford University Press
198 Madison Avenue, New York, NY 10016, United States of America.

Library of Congress Cataloging-in-Publication Data
Names: Galea, Sandro, author.
Title: The contagion next time / Sandro Galea.
Description: New York, NY : Oxford University Press, [2022] |
Includes bibliographical references and index.
Identifiers: LCCN 2021038471 (print) | LCCN 2021038472 (ebook) |
ISBN 9780197576427 (hardback) | ISBN 9780197576441 (epub) |
ISBN 9780197576458
Subjects: MESH: Health Status Disparities | Social Determinants of Health |
Global Health | Socioeconomic Factors | Delivery of Health Care |
Pandemics—prevention & control | COVID-19 | United States
Classification: LCC RA563.M56 (print) | LCC RA563.M56 (ebook) |
NLM WA 300 AA1 | DDC 362.1089—dc23
LC record available at https://lccn.loc.gov/2021038471
LC ebook record available at https://lccn.loc.gov/2021038472

DOI: 10.1093/oso/9780197576427.001.0001

1 3 5 7 9 8 6 4 2

Printed by Sheridan Books, Inc., United States of America

This book is dedicated, as always, to Isabel Tess Galea, Oliver Luke Galea, and Dr. Margaret Kruk

All I maintain is that on this earth there are pestilences and there are victims, and it's up to us, so far as possible, not to join forces with the pestilences.

—Albert Camus, *The Plague*

You don't command wind in the direction it blows, but you command a ship in the direction it sails.

—Matshona Dhliwayo

Contents

Acknowledgments

This book emerges from conversations throughout 2020 that often centered around what that unprecedented year meant for our present, and what it meant for the world we wish to build. I am deeply grateful to all with whom I had the privilege of engaging in conversation throughout the year. A central acknowledgment to Eric DelGizzo and Catherine Ettman. For years now, our triumvirate has been the bedrock of my writing, creating space for ideas to be tested, shaped, improved. Eric's hand is here felt in every page of this book. He has an extraordinary ability to inhabit my thoughts, sharpen them, hone them, and put them in historical and Shakespearean perspective. This book, and much else of my public writing, could not happen without him. Thank you. Catherine's pragmatic and principled eye on what we are trying to do—and why we are doing it—keeps the three of us grounded, pulls us back from occasional overdigression, and reminds me again and again of what a privilege it is to be able to write for a living. Full credit for rendering the figures that illustrate this book, and for bringing to visual life ideas that were only abstractions, goes to Kappy Arnold. Conversations with Drs. Nason Maani, Salma Abdalla, and Margaret Kruk, many of the latter taking place during weekend morning runs, helped me sort, filter, and organize thoughts about what we were living through in 2020, giving me the on-ramp to the ideas that became this book. I owe a debt of gratitude to Sarah Humphreville, my editor at Oxford University Press, who immediately saw the potential of these ideas and encouraged me to turn them into this book, nurturing it to completion. And, finally, I am grateful to all—too many to name—with whom I had the privilege of writing other academic and public pieces during the past year. I have learned from each of you, and the ideas developed in those pieces shaped my thinking, leading to this book. Thank you.

Introduction

It began with a cough.

A member of the coronavirus family, the virus produced symptoms that included high fever, dry cough, body aches, diarrhea, and pneumonia. It spread primarily through respiratory droplets emitted when an infected person coughed or sneezed. This made it important to minimize person-to-person contact and observe social distancing in public spaces where the virus could be transmitted.

Once the world became aware of the disease, it mobilized to stop it. These efforts were successful. Quarantine measures, quickly adopted, substantially slowed the spread of the disease. Within months of the detection of the virus in humans, the World Health Organization (WHO) declared the outbreak contained. A total of 8,098 people were infected during the outbreak, and 774 died.

I am speaking, of course, of the 2003 SARS outbreak, although one could be forgiven for initially thinking I meant Covid-19, the virus that was first detected in late 2019 and which became a global pandemic. The SARS outbreak had much in common with Covid-19. Both were caused by coronaviruses. They shared symptoms and means of transmission. Yet SARS was contained quickly, with relatively few infections and deaths, while Covid-19 became a global crisis that infected and killed millions, and effectively made the earth stand still.

Why did Covid-19 do so much while SARS did comparatively little? The answer is in large part luck, good and bad. A feature of Covid-19 was that its viral load tended to peak early in the course of infection, before the development of major symptoms, so people with the virus could spread it before even knowing they were sick. Viral loads for SARS peaked later, so one could know one had the disease, and self-isolate, before posing maximum risk to others. Were it not for this difference, we might have seen a pandemic on the scale of Covid-19 nearly two decades before this challenge ultimately emerged. And it could even have been worse. SARS is much deadlier than Covid-19. Had it matched or exceeded the infectiousness of Covid-19, the world might still be reeling from the consequences.

So we got lucky that Covid-19 was not worse than it was, and we were unlucky that features of Covid-19 facilitated its rapid spread. And, as we shall discuss further in this book, to end the spread of Covid-19 we had the good fortune of seeing the extraordinary success of one particular approach—vaccination—emerge quickly, saving us from a much longer and more devastating pandemic. But, I suggest, the key question we should be asking ourselves, as we reflect on the pandemic, on how much worse it could have been, and on how much worse a future pandemic can be, is this: what challenges were facing us when SARS hit that we should have tended to so that we could have handled Covid-19 better? And, by extension, what are the challenges we should tend to now to avoid the contagion next time?

Before continuing, I should note what I mean when I say "we." Covid-19 was a global crisis, and preventing pandemics is ultimately a global responsibility. However, in addressing Covid-19, each country had its own unique failures and successes. I realize as I am writing that this book will come to life at a time when the pandemic remains an active concern in many parts of the world. I am writing from within American public health, and my aim in this book is centrally to address how we can improve health in an American context. At the same time, we are all global citizens, the forces that shape health transcend borders, and health in the United States is inextricably linked to health in the wider world. For this reason, while the "we" of this book refers to us in the United States, our global context will never be far from the discussion, particularly in the book's early chapters, as we take a wider view of the pandemic, before focusing more specifically on how it unfolded in America.

This book makes the argument that we have, for many decades, let challenges grow and accumulate, until Covid-19 meant we could no longer look away. When Covid-19 emerged, we were about five decades deep into a period of neglecting the foundational forces that shape health, and this neglect made us vulnerable to the pandemic. These forces are the focus of this book.

These forces are perhaps best introduced by way of metaphor. Imagine you are on a ship, passing through a violent storm. There were warnings of rough weather before the ship left port; even so, the storm feels sudden, unexpected. Fortunately, the ship is crewed by experienced sailors who know what to do. This is not their first storm. They act coolly in the crisis, attending to their tasks with a sense of urgency that never gives way to panic. Although the winds and rain make it hard for you to get your bearings, the crew have a very clear sense of where their vessel is headed. With the use of their instruments, they are able to quickly regain course when the storm threatens to divert them. But there are moments when the way is not so clear and the captain must make a judgment call about what to do next. Supported by her team, guided by her knowledge of the sea, she is able to make the decisions that bring the vessel through the storm and safely to port.

The story need not have ended this way, of course. If any element of crew, captain, or ship had been altered, the outcome could have been less favorable. If the sailors had lacked experience, they might not have had the resilience under pressure to adapt to challenge. If they had been less sure of where the voyage was headed, they could have been easily thrown off course. If their captain had mishandled her decisions, she could have led her crew to the bottom of the sea. If all these unwelcome elements were in place at once, the fate of the ship would have been sealed before it ever set sail.

This was the state of our "ship" when Covid-19 struck. The captain was our political leadership; the sailors were us, the people, and how healthy we were; the conditions of the ship itself were the conditions of where we live, work, and play; and the destination of the vessel was our broader approach to health. At the level of political leadership, our response to the crisis was patchy at best. In the United States, the chaotic and conflicting approach of the Trump administration hindered the federal government's ability to coordinate action. As for our health, when the pandemic hit we were far less healthy than we could and should have been had we paid attention to creating the healthiest possible population. And as for the ship itself, the pandemic happened in a context of disinvestment in the systems that support health at the population level. I mean not only individual organizations such as the Centers for Disease Control and Prevention (CDC) but also the network of policies and institutions that create the conditions for health to flourish. This includes environmental protections, the conditions of our neighborhoods, our social safety net, and investment in ameliorating the socioeconomic inequities that create poor health.

Our disinvestment in these structures reflects how our approach to health—the direction of our ship—has been misguided. We tend to think of health mainly in terms of doctors and medicines. But doctors and medicines are not health; they are where we turn when health eludes us, in the hope they can make us better. Health is the state of not being sick to begin with, and it is shaped by social, economic, environmental, and political forces. We do not generally think of these forces when we think about health, and they certainly do not guide our health spending. We invest vast amounts of money in healthcare, but comparatively little in health. We have been moving in the wrong direction when it comes to health, and while recent years have seen the beginning of a shift toward greater focus on the forces that shape health, Covid-19 emerged in a context where we were still broadly conflating health with healthcare and neglecting the true causes of health.

This book is about how we can address these foundational forces in order to build a better ship. It will focus primarily on the crew (our health), the ship (the infrastructure of policies and resources that support our health), the direction of the vessel (the values that inform our pursuit of health), and the politics that informs all of this. I argue throughout this book that we—not just Americans, but all global citizens—have an opportunity now, in the wake of Covid-19, to address the vulnerabilities the virus exposed, to create the world we should have created after SARS, one where pandemics cannot emerge. To have healthier sailors, to build a better ship, and to sail in a direction that leads to health.

Of course, the challenge of the Covid-19 moment was not just the challenge of a pandemic. The time of the coronavirus saw multiple crises. Covid-19 quickly led to an economic downturn, as the lockdown measures taken to slow the disease caused a level of unemployment not seen since the Great Depression. Many workers who kept their jobs faced uncertainty over when or whether their next paycheck would come. Then, on May 25, 2020, an African American man named George Floyd was killed during an encounter with a white police officer who knelt on Floyd's neck for nearly nine minutes while he struggled to breathe. A video of the encounter sparked widespread protests, civil unrest, and an international reckoning with the issues of racism and police brutality. Taken together, these difficulties created a moment of crisis unprecedented in recent decades.

In earlier times, the sudden emergence of such overlapping challenges might have been interpreted as supernatural—divine punishment for a society gone astray. We do not think this way anymore
because we can see how these challenges represent an accumulation
of societal shortcomings that all conspired in 2020 to surface problems
that we have long neglected—pushing us, I hope, to address issues
we should have addressed many decades ago. Consider the death of
George Floyd. At first there may seem to be little connection between
an isolated case of police violence and the forces that shaped the
Covid-19 crisis. Looking closer, however, we can see how Floyd's
death occurred in a context of historical injustice, rooted in the legacy
of slavery, that has caused Black Americans to suffer a disproportionate
burden of poor health. This inequity was clear during the pandemic,
as Black Americans were likelier to get sick and die from the disease
than whites, a health gap consistent with our history. From residential segregation to mass incarceration, maternal mortality, and everyday
incidents of racism, including police brutality, Black Americans suffer
from poorer health.

The protests that followed the death of George Floyd, with their
calls for an end to racism and systems of injustice, were reactions to
the same conditions that create poor health in our society, conditions
that helped Covid-19 to spread. These conditions were also expressed
in the economic shock of that time. Just as the United States has structural divides that unfold along the lines of race, it has divides shaped by
economic inequality. Money is one of the most robust determinants
of health; those who have it are likelier to live longer, healthier lives
than those who do not. This is reflected in the nearly fourteen-year
gap in life expectancy between the richest and poorest Americans. This
is the context in which the economic difficulties caused by Covid-19
unfolded. When the disease struck the United States, it intersected
with the already vulnerable health of low-income populations, a vulnerability worsened by lost wages and unemployment caused by the
virus. As with race, the economic divides in our society made the work
of the virus far easier than it might have been, exposing us all to greater
risk of contagion.

It is important to stress that none of this is new. Covid-19 was a
novel coronavirus, but the structural vulnerabilities that allowed it
to take hold extend far back. Racial and economic injustices have
been with us since the beginning of the United States itself, as has

the poor health these problems create. The pandemic represented a new interplay of these foundational forces, just as each storm is a new combination of wind and rain. It is our responsibility to engage with foundational issues that leave us vulnerable to novel health threats, to ensure our vessel can withstand whatever comes. Each storm is different, but the sailors, captain, and crew of the ship are the same, and we need to make sure they are in proper order, for our voyage to be as smooth as it can be.

Racism, marginalization, socioeconomic inequality—our failure to address these forces is what left us vulnerable to Covid-19, allowing the disease to grow into the crisis it became. Had we tackled these challenges twenty years ago, after the outbreak of SARS, we might have created a world where Covid-19 could have been quickly contained. Instead, we allowed our ship to drift off course.

We have not yet faced the perfect storm. As bad as Covid-19 was, it was not as terrible as it could have been. But the perfect storm is coming. Novel viruses will continue to emerge. And we should be ready. Unless we address the foundational forces that underlie health, nothing we do will sufficiently prepare us for the next pandemic. This is a hard truth to face, particularly now that we have largely emerged from the shadow of Covid-19. There is always the temptation to feel our work is done once we have navigated a crisis. We want to move forward and are hesitant to revisit past trauma. This is understandable, but it is not the way to create a healthier world. We may think that, having just come out of one crisis, we will be able to muddle through the next, even if it is worse than what came before. But the best way to navigate a future crisis is to ensure it never occurs. This means learning the lessons of the past. We must have the wisdom to be not just reactive but reflective. We must address the most urgent question to emerge from Covid-19: how can we stop something like this from ever happening again?

This book is meant as a reflection on the Covid-19 moment, bringing to the surface lessons that emerged over the course of the pandemic. It is about the foundations of health in our society and how we can strengthen them to prevent the next outbreak from becoming a pandemic. It is not a book about how to create vaccines, invent new treatments, or shore up public health departments such as the CDC. These are all necessary steps, worthy of books of their own. But they do not address health on the deepest level: that of politics, culture, economics, and the values that inform how we approach these forces.

No one could have predicted that a pandemic would strike when it did, nor could we have known precisely how it would intersect with our world when it arrived. But we did know that a pandemic would strike sooner or later. It was indeed possible to imagine that vulnerabilities in the state of our health would amplify the danger of an outbreak whenever one occurred. That the interplay of virus and vulnerabilities almost immediately informed three massive challenges—disease, economic shock, and civil unrest—suggests the importance of foundational forces and the degree to which our neglect of them has made our position precarious.

I have spent my career writing and thinking about these forces. I have written previously about them in my last book, *Well: What We Need to Talk About When We Talk About Health*. The aim of this book now is to show how they intersected with Covid-19, and why our experience of the pandemic makes engaging with these forces that much more important. The first section of the book will address the current state of our country, world, and health. In many ways it is a better and healthier time to be alive than ever before. Yet the presence of deep inequities keeps us from being as healthy as we could be, or as prepared for the next pandemic. The second section will address the foundational forces that shape health and how we can engage with them to build a healthier world. These include the spaces where we live, work, and play, and the influence of politics, power, and money. As we engage with these forces, our work should be guided by compassion, a desire for social and economic justice, and a recognition that health is a public good. These values are the subject of the third section. The final section will address how science can inform our pursuit of a healthier world, how we can work within complexity and doubt, maintaining humility, with an eye toward what matters most for health.

I will discuss foundational forces to illustrate how they shaped Covid-19, so we can understand them better as we prepare for the next contagion. I will focus on health as a public good because, to my mind, our failure to see health this way led to many of the problems we faced during Covid-19. Unless we think of health as a public good, we will be unable to do right by the world between now and the next outbreak. And I will talk about science because it plays a critical role in informing the actions we must take, at the level of policy and elsewhere, to build a healthier world.

The sum total of the Covid-19 pandemic may have been unprecedented, but its component parts were deeply familiar. As it spread, it exploited health gaps that have been with us for decades—centuries, in the case of American racial inequities. In the same way, the observations and recommendations of this book may feel familiar, but they amount to an argument we do not often hear, and which is, I think, radical in its implications: Creating a world that is no longer vulnerable to pandemics means creating a healthy world. Creating a healthy world means making the changes, at the structural level, that will prevent the contagion next time. Absent this fundamental change, it will not matter what else we do—we will still be vulnerable to pandemics. It will not matter how cutting-edge our treatments are, how nimble our process of vaccine development, how sophisticated our disease surveillance. All this is necessary, but it is not sufficient. We need to do what we did not do after SARS and invest in creating the conditions for health, guided by science and informed by our values.

In 2017, *Time* ran a cover story titled "Warning: We Are Not Ready for the Next Pandemic." Despite widespread understanding that we were indeed not ready, we did not make the changes that had to happen to be ready for a challenge like Covid-19. As with SARS, it was a feature of the disease itself—in this case its relative lack of lethality—that saved us from the worst-case scenario. It may seem strange to say the crisis of Covid-19 was not the worst-case scenario, given the damage it was able to do, but the characterization is correct. It was not the deadliest contagion we could have faced—but the next pandemic may be. And the disquieting fact is that *Time* could easily run its 2017 headline today. We are still not ready for the next pandemic. But we can be—we must be. This book aims to help us get there.

THE CONTAGION
NEXT TIME

SECTION 1

The World We Live In

I

A Better and Healthier Time
to Be Alive than Ever

In April 2020, the United Nations University World Institute for Development Economics Research released a working paper estimating that the economic consequences of the Covid-19 pandemic could drive up to half a billion people around the world into poverty. This worst-case scenario was significant for many reasons. Clearly it brought home again the horrors of the pandemic. But the data also show the first increase in global poverty since 1990. This reflects something paradoxical about the Covid-19 moment. On one hand, it felt like a time of unprecedented disruption. From the pandemic itself to its economic effects and the global unrest over racial injustice with which the pandemic intersected, it felt as if the world was experiencing a time of historically unique challenge. On the other hand, that an increase in global poverty could be seen as such a profound anomaly speaks to the fact that when the pandemic appeared, in many respects the world had never been better off or healthier. In a number of key areas—life expectancy, rises in education and literacy, reductions in preventable diseases such as HIV/AIDS—the twenty-first century was, and is, a more favorable time to be alive than any other point in recorded history.

I realize it is unorthodox to start a book about a pandemic by talking about positives. But I do so to set the groundwork for how we can create a better world that is resistant to future pandemics, to show what we have done, and to argue that there is much more we can do. In this post-Covid-19 moment, it can be easy to overlook our historical successes. In our daily lives, what is going wrong tends to come into view more readily than what is going right. The news and social media bring us a constant stream of tragedies and injustices. On any given day, we are likelier to hear a news anchor report that thirty-seven people were killed in a terrorist attack than we are to hear her say that global poverty continued to decline, as it has for the last thirty years. Yet news of the decline in global poverty is far more representative of the trajectory of life for most people in the twenty-first century than news of a terrorist attack is. Seeing this requires us to look beyond the moment, when our feelings about our health are clouded by the remaining soupy fog of Covid-19 memories, and view the sweep of history, seeing how the decades leading up to now have ushered in unparalleled progress.

This chapter is an attempt to present this perspective. I am starting a book about the global pandemic with a look at how healthy we had become, aiming to help us understand the forces that shape health and to show us how to engage with them to prevent another pandemic. Seeing the scale of the progress we have made in building a healthier world raises a question about the drivers of this success. What are the factors that make the difference between health and disease in populations? When we have answers to these questions, we can apply them to yet another question: what must we do to build an even healthier world, one that is no longer vulnerable to pandemics?

A good way to find these answers is by looking at the last century. How our past shaped our present holds lessons for how we might shape our future. Exploring the difference between epochs can shed light on the forces that influence the lives and health of successive generations.

So how does life in the first year of the twentieth century compare to now? In some respects, discussing 1900 and discussing today is like talking about two different worlds. There are many ways to measure this difference, from advances in transportation (horse and buggy at the start of the twentieth century, space travel by the end of it) to progress in communication (the age of the telegraph giving way to the telephone, television, computer, and internet). But among the most striking measures of progress is the rise in life expectancy. In the United States, a child born in 1900 could on average expect to live to about age forty-seven. Today, that child can expect to live to about age seventy-nine. Can you imagine how different your life would be if you expected to live to your mid-forties compared to expecting to live to your late seventies? All manner of choices that follow, including, for example, getting married later or getting a graduate degree, simply would not have been likely without this change in our health, our longer lives.

Why this difference? The answer most people would give is simple: better medicine. It is a compelling answer, but it is only partially true—very partially. Medicine matters, but it is part of a broader network of factors that shape our health. In this context, the role of medicine is quite minor. This is reflected by the rise in life expectancy during the last century. One of the reasons life expectancy is among the most useful measures of overall population health is because no single factor accounts for it. Life expectancy is the product of the context in which our lives unfold. It is this context that is most responsible for health. So while it is true that the last century saw remarkable achievements in medicine—from polio vaccination to, more recently, advanced treatments for HIV/AIDS—medicine alone cannot account for such a significant, multidecade gain in life expectancy. Something deeper is at work.

Let us, then, compare the life of someone born in 1900 with the life of someone born today. In the years leading up to 1900, the United States industrialized and urbanized in the wake of the Civil War. Concurrent with these trends came waves of immigrants hoping to settle in this land of rapidly growing opportunity. They came for better lives, yet for many the opportunity of America was interwoven with hardship. Immigrants in cities such as New York often found themselves living in squalid, overcrowded tenements of the sort documented by Jacob Riis in his 1890 book, *How the Other Half Lives: Studies Among the Tenements of New York*. The photographs in the book expose the network of slums to which poverty consigned scores of immigrants.

Such conditions bred injury and disease; of particular, poignant note were their consequences for the health and development of children. When children are abused, are malnourished, or lack quality education, this ripples through the rest of life, creating a pattern of poor health. In addition to facing such conditions in urban slums, many children of that era worked dangerous jobs to help support their families. This was a time before widespread worker protections and child labor laws in the United States. While some reforms were being adopted even then, young workers could still be exploited by employers who had little care for their safety. At every turn, the health of the young was threatened by this confluence of social, economic, and political factors, which made their lives a struggle.

Imagine, then, a child is born in 1900 to immigrant parents in New York City. His parents are poor, lacking money for basic amenities, including clean clothes and nutritious food. Like so many immigrant families, they live in cheap, overcrowded tenement housing, where necessities such as electricity and proper ventilation are hard to come by. In this environment, the boy is often malnourished and sick. Later, instead of getting a good education, he begins working odd jobs to earn extra money for his family. They are dangerous jobs, which result in the child sustaining a number of injuries. With the outbreak of World War I, he sees military service as both a patriotic duty and a way out of poverty. At sixteen, he lies about his age in order to enlist, seeing combat in the final year of the war, which leaves him with a case of what was then called shell shock but which we now call post-traumatic stress disorder (PTSD).

After the war, he returns home, but his PTSD continues to make life difficult for him. He eventually establishes himself as a grocer, working his way up to a managerial position. He starts to dream of buying his own store, but then the United States is suddenly hit with the economic shock of the Great Depression, which leaves him penniless and unemployed. These challenges worsen his mental health struggles, and he begins to drink heavily. All this leads to him passing away in his early forties from the effects of alcoholism, despair, and a lifetime of injury and poor health.

Were we to meet this man near the end of his life, we would likely ascribe his decline to a series of poor choices on his part and perhaps to his lack of access to adequate healthcare. But when we examine the full range of his experience, we see how his poor health was more fundamentally a product of the historical moment in which he lived. Poverty, urbanization, poor housing, inability to access education and nutritious food, lack of a social safety net and legal protections for workers, war, and economic crisis all created a context for poor health to emerge. These forces were at the heart of Americans' lower life expectancy at the start of the twentieth century. The same forces are just as influential in our own time, but the nature of their influence has changed as conditions have improved.

Let us consider a child born in the United States more recently—say, in 1990. At that time, the world had just emerged from the Cold

War and was enjoying a sense of optimism about the future. The US economy was doing well, and there was a feeling that the global catastrophes of the twentieth century were, with the approach of the new millennium, something humanity had perhaps outgrown. This is the context in which the child is born. She grows up in a middle-class household. Her family is not rich, but they have enough so that she never lacks food, clothes, or other basic necessities. Naturally, this means her home has electricity, adequate space, and, later on, internet access. While she works summer jobs as a teen and young adult, she does so for pocket money, not from a need to support her family. She attends college and quickly transitions to a professional career as a doctor. She marries, has three kids, and currently lives a comfortable life in New Jersey, where she enjoys multiple hobbies in her spare time, takes yearly vacations, and suffers from no major health issues.

The contrast between her life and that of the child born in 1900 is stark. The child in 1900 had a future clouded by disadvantage, making a healthy life difficult for him to attain. Yet for the child born in 1990, having a healthy life seemed a relatively straightforward matter, a path of unbroken progress from birth to her adult life in New Jersey. But this path was straightforward only because the state of the world in the last thirty years made it so. Lack of large-scale, global conflict meant many young people could grow up without facing the trauma of war. A strong economy meant more people could access the basic resources necessary for health. The internet democratized access to information, supplementing the education available in public schools. Networks of legal protections for workers made jobs less dangerous than they were a hundred years ago. If the child born in 1990 had needed it, there was a social safety net in place to help her through hard times. And, of course, an American woman in today's world can vote, which she would not have been able to do nationally before 1920. As we will discuss more deeply in later chapters, health is closely linked to politics. Exclusion from the political process undermines health, as do the marginalization and denial of dignity reflected by this shutting out.

These changes, far more than any medical innovations, account for improvements in health and life expectancy. It is true that between 1900 and 1990 tremendous advances were made in the field of medicine. Had the child born in 1990 become sick, she would have had access to better treatments than the child born in 1900. But more significant for health were the changes in how we live our lives, changes that were shaped by social, economic, and political forces. Health means not needing medicine because we do not become sick in the first place. Whether we get sick in the first place depends largely on our quality of life and the forces that shape it. The influence of these forces is like air—easy to overlook precisely because it is so ubiquitous. It is what we encounter each day, with direct implications for the health of our bodies and minds.

The child born in 1990 can be forgiven for not always appreciating her luck at being born into such favorable conditions for health, because these conditions are so much a part of her life she does not need to notice them. She is not alone in this. How often do any of us start the day by noting our good fortune to be living amid conditions that are far healthier than those of a hundred years ago? How often do we pause to take stock of how abundant nutritious food is compared to past eras, or to recognize that quality education, while still not available to all, is within reach of so many? Yet if the child born in 1900 traveled by time machine to the present day, he would likely be astounded by how much better everything has become, by and large.

The advantage of time travel, of course, is that it would make unavoidably clear the effect of foundational forces on the lives and health of successive generations. Seen in real time, these forces can be subtle and easy to miss. But there are times when their influence converges at precise historical moments to draw a sharp line between good health and bad. When these moments arise, no special insight is necessary to see that events are being steered by large-scale forces. Covid-19 was such a moment. It was a time when everyone could see how politics, the economy, racial injustice, new technologies, and shifting ideas of national and global solidarity intersected to shape health. Even as we pursued medical solutions to the crisis, this broader context was never far from mind.

During Covid-19, it was jarring to realize that something as intimate as our health could be so much at the mercy of seemingly abstract forces. In a sense, it was akin to feeling the influence of such forces during wartime, when their effect on health is arguably most direct. Wartime is also when the line is clearest between generations who are able to easily experience good health and those whose path to health is thorny. If you are a young person living during a time of global war, you are likelier to face premature injury and death than a young person living in a time of relative peace. In this context, medicine makes scant difference. Compared with the hazards of war—including war's effects on civilian populations, in the form of starvation, displacement, and death—the quality of drugs available in the field hospital matters relatively little. Of greater importance are the forces that lead soldiers to the fight in the first place. As anyone who has studied the history of war—particularly that of World War I—knows, wars tend to begin because of a complex interplay of historical, social, economic, and technological factors. These factors underlie the risk run by every soldier who has ever faced enemy fire. Such factors may fade into the background in the heat of battle, when survival seems a matter of skill, luck, and individual decision-making. Nevertheless, the reason these elements come into play at all is that global conditions reached a point at a given historical period where war became a fact of life for everyone alive at that time. Differences over the years in education, employment safety, housing, availability of nutritious food, and the existence of social programs are no less important in shaping the health of each generation than the forces that decide whether that generation will experience peace or war. And all of these forces ultimately emerge from the same place—the convergence of politics, economics, culture, and other foundational forces.

In the years since 1900, there have been, tragically, many wars all over the world. Yet the historical forces with which these conflicts converged ultimately shaped an era that is healthier than ever before. Global average life expectancy has more than doubled since 1900. This reflects an upward trend in life expectancy that began in early-industrializing countries around the start of the nineteenth century and unfolded in other parts of the world in the mid-nineteenth century. While inequalities in life expectancy persist by region, all parts of the world have seen an increase in average life span in the last 150 years (Figure 1.1).

What is the reason for this rise in life expectancy? Broadly speaking, the answer is better living standards generated by the social, political, and industrial trends that drive global economic development. The unfolding of these trends over the last 150 years has helped lower the cost of goods and broaden access to the funds that purchase them. It is a simple calculation. Health depends on our ability to access the basic resources that allow us to live and thrive. These resources cost money. The cheaper they are, the more easily we will be able to buy them, and the healthier we will be.

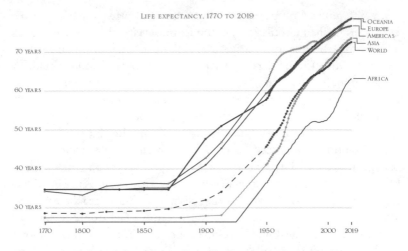

Figure 1.1. Adapted from figure found at Roser M, Ortiz-Ospina E, Ritchie H. Life Expectancy. Our World in Data website. https:// ourworldindata.org/life-expectancy. Published 2013. Updated October 2019. Accessed December 31, 2020. Licensed under CC BY 4.0.
Figure data were compiled by Our World in Data from estimates by Riley JC, Clio Infra, and the United Nations Population Division. Data published in the following sources: Riley JC. Estimates of Regional and Global Life Expectancy, 1800–2001. *Population and Development Review.* 2005; 31(3): 537–543. Zijdeman R, Ribeira da Silva F. Life Expectancy at Birth (Total). http://hdl.handle.net/10622/LKYT53. IISH Dataverse, V1. 2015. UN Population Division: 2019. https://population.un.org/wpp/Download/ Standard/Population/.

Figure 1.1 is a clear illustration of this, showing that life expectancy began a significant increase around the middle of the nineteenth century. This coincided with the quickening pace of the Industrial Revolution, as economic systems became based on mechanization and living standards began to rise around the world. It is perhaps a cliché to say "A rising tide lifts all boats," but during this period the tide was indeed rising, and millions were seeing the benefits in better health and longer lives.

Before going further, it is important to note that economic development is by no means a panacea. All boats may rise, but rarely at the same pace. Just as economic growth can drive progress, it can also fuel persistent inequalities within populations. This is true across countries and economic systems. As we see in Figure 1.1, while global life expectancy has risen over the last 150 years, there are still inequalities among the beneficiaries of this progress. Economic development is a power-ful engine for creating better living standards, but it can also exclude some people from accessing its benefits. These inequalities are a central challenge for health; addressing them is core to building the healthiest possible world, one that is no longer vulnerable to pandemics. I will discuss inequalities at greater length in Chapter 2.

It is also important to acknowledge another caveat to the progress of the last 150 years. The environmental destruction that has emerged as a byproduct of global economic development has created one of the most pressing threats to health that we collectively face: climate change. Our industrialized economy has taken a toll on the planet, including its temperature and weather systems, and these changes threaten us in both the near and long term. In recent years, this challenge has taken the form of more frequent and more severe natural disasters—hurricanes, earthquakes, mudslides, and droughts. The consequences of accelerating climate change will become direr if we do not take steps now to address the problem. Climate change is not a primary focus of this book, but it will undoubtedly dominate our thinking in the com-ing decades—and it should—as we look to build a healthier world.

But climate change, inequalities, and our concern for the pop-ulations most affected by these challenges do not negate the truth, reflected across the centuries, that global economic development has likely done more for health than any medicine we have yet devised. The child born in 1900 was still fairly near the beginning of this pro-cess of development, yet even he enjoyed greater health and material resources than a child born 130 years earlier, when life expectancy was below forty years in the Americas and closer to thirty in other parts of the world. Even though the life of the child born in 1900 was in many ways more difficult than that of the child born in 1990, he still enjoyed advantages brought about by the economic changes of his era. We can imagine his immigrant parents still living in their former country, experiencing poverty and persecution, lacking options, but hearing of America, with its plentiful job opportunities and the chance it afforded to rise in the world—or, at least, to build a life where one's children could rise—and being drawn to its shores. Once in the United States, this family may have lived a life that, while looking almost impossibly hardscrabble when seen through the lens of the intervening century, could well have exceeded their wildest dreams. Housing may have been cramped, but at least it was adequate, and—compared to life in places beyond the city—modern. Jobs may have been dangerous, but at least there *were* jobs. Their income may not have matched the wealth of a Rockefeller, or even that of a middle-class American today, but at least there was income to be had, and some savings to be accrued. Taken together, these conditions were by no means perfect, but they were better than they had been, and they continued to get better as the century progressed, as did the health these conditions shaped.

This raises an important point, one worth bearing in mind throughout the discussions in this book. The following chapters address how we can improve health by focusing on the systems that underlie our society. Often, these systems are aligned in ways that challenge health, creating a status quo that excludes certain populations from the resources necessary to live healthy lives. This is possible because we have collectively accepted the status quo. The first step toward better health, then, is choosing to no longer accept the conditions that undermine it at the structural level. However, in making the critique that helps us to see these conditions and take steps to improve them, we should also acknowledge there is much about the status quo that is good and makes us healthier, and that the structures that support these advances should be left intact. The general trend of the last 150 years has been toward better collective quality of life and better health. Certainly, not all have shared this progress equally, and addressing this will be central to the steps suggested by this book. But it is also true that creating a healthier world does not require us to dismantle all that came before, much of which is responsible for our healthier present. Rather, we need to be discerning in our efforts to create a healthier world, and build on the progress we have made while addressing the challenges we still face.

One of the key markers of this progress is the one that began this chapter—the decline in extreme poverty, roughly defined as the number of people living on less than $1.90 per day. In the last two centuries, the proportion of people living in extreme poverty has significantly decreased (Figure 1.2).

Declines in poverty were fundamental to the creation of the healthier world we now enjoy. Poverty is a core driver of poor health because it reflects an acute lack of the resources necessary for health. To live in poverty is often to be excluded from access to the food, clean water, clothing, sanitation, shelter, and educational opportunities that make health possible. Poverty is intergenerational, keeping families locked

WORLD POPULATION LIVING IN EXTREME POVERTY, 1820–2015

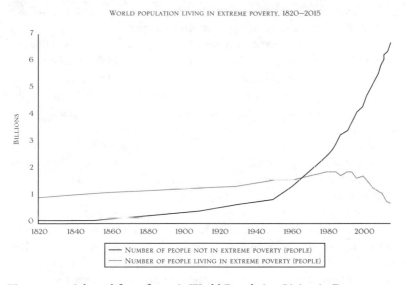

Figure 1.2. Adapted from figure in World Population Living in Extreme Poverty, 1820–2015. Our World in Data website. https://ourworldindata .org/grapher/world-population-in-extreme-poverty-absolute. Accessed December 31, 2020. Licensed under CC BY 4.0. Based on visualization found in Ravallion M. *The Economics of Poverty: History, Measurement, and Policy.* Oxford, UK: Oxford University Press; 2016. Poverty estimates 1981 and later taken from World Bank's PovcalNet, iresearch.worldbank .org/PovcalNet/. Data from 1980 and earlier taken from Bourguignon F, Morrisson C. Inequality Among World Citizens: 1820–1992. *American Economic Review.* 92 (4): 727–744. Absolute number of world population from Our World in Data website, world population data set: https:// ourworldindata.org/world-population-growth.

in cycles of disadvantage, as the challenges faced by parents limit the options of their children. And it is often children who suffer most from poverty, as the conditions into which they are born create levels of deprivation that threaten health at each stage of development. According to UNICEF, approximately 385 million children live in extreme poverty. This number is still far too high—any number would be—but the progress we have made in reducing the number of children in extreme poverty remains a key element of the progress we have made so far in building a healthier world.

It makes sense that as extreme poverty has declined, we have also seen a rise in the ability of populations to access the resources money can buy, resources necessary for health. Take food, for example. Food is one of those resources we sometimes overlook until we experience the lack of it. The rise in living standards of our era coupled with persistent inequalities has meant that while many people are able to live their whole lives without doubting the availability of the next meal, others must live without ever once feeling this confidence. Fortunately, the number of people in the latter category has declined in the last thirty years. Despite recent upticks, the number of people who are undernourished has fallen from about 1 billion people in 1991 to about 820 million in 2017 (Figure 1.3).

Another indicator of our world becoming a healthier place is the steep decline in child mortality. The deaths of children used to occur with tragic regularity. Some estimates suggest that in 1800, parents lost an average of two to three children in the early years of life. Child mortality was common enough to be a central theme in art and literature, notably in the work of Charles Dickens. In our own time, about 15,000 children die each day. It is hard to suggest that such a number could represent any kind of progress—as with child poverty, any child mortality rate that is not zero should be unacceptable to us. But the fact is that from 1800 to 1950, global child mortality fell from 43 percent to 22.5 percent. This progress was initially confined mostly to wealthier counties; in 1950, child mortality remained high in counties where the resources necessary for health were less widely distributed than elsewhere. In the years since, however, declines in child mortality have become closer to universal, with reductions in Asia, Africa, and Latin America, not just in the European countries where much of this progress was once concentrated. Child mortality rates in these regions are now much closer to where rates in Europe were in the 1950s, suggesting a hopeful trajectory (Figure 1.4).

For much of the high-income world, the prospect of losing a child is unthinkable. The fact that it is unthinkable reflects the progress we have made in creating a healthier world. By improving the conditions that shape health, we were able to turn what was once a common tragedy into something so rare that it has become difficult for many to even imagine. Another place where we have achieved this is in the area of maternal mortality. Death during childbirth was once not uncommon. In nineteenth-century Finland, for example, maternal mortality

GLOBAL NUMBER OF PEOPLE WHO ARE UNDERNOURISHED

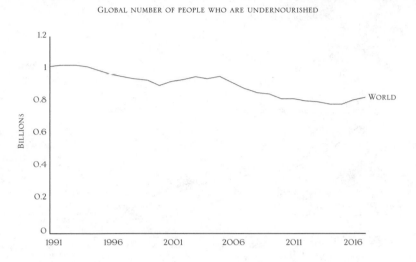

Figure 1.3. Adapted from figure found at Roser M, Ritchie H. Hunger and Undernourishment. Our World in Data website. https://ourworldindata.org/hunger-and-undernourishment. Accessed December 31, 2020. Licensed under CC BY 4.0. Data prior to 2005 was generated using the following sources: The Prevalence of Undernourishment. World Bank, World Development Indicators. https://data.worldbank.org/indicator. FAO, IFAD, UNICEF, WFP, WHO. *The State of Food Security and Nutrition in the World 2017: Building Resilience for Peace and Food Security.* Rome: FAO; 2017. Global population figures from the UN FAO database. Data from 2005 and after were generated using FAO, IFAD, UNICEF, WFP, WHO. *The State of Food Security and Nutrition in the World 2018: Building Climate Resilience for Food Security and Nutrition.* Rome: FAO; 2018.

was between 800 and 1,000 deaths per 100,000 births, amounting to about a 0.9 percent chance of death during childbirth in a country where women at that time gave birth to an average of five children. Thanks largely to advances in hospital sanitation, this risk has declined significantly, and mothers giving birth in Finland now have just a 0.003 percent chance of death (Figure 1.5).

We can see declines in maternal mortality throughout the world, reflecting improvements in the conditions in which women live and give birth. There is still much work to be done, particularly in addressing the disparities that concentrate so many maternal deaths

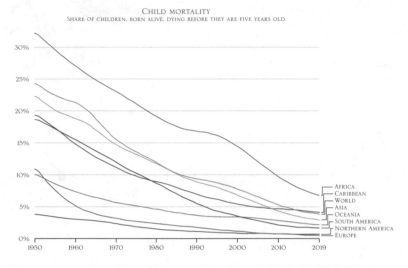

Figure 1.4. Adapted from figure found at Roser M, Ritchie H, Dadonaite B. Child and Infant Mortality. Our World in Data website. https://ourworldindata.org/child-mortality. Published 2013. Updated November 2019. Accessed December 31, 2020. Licensed under CC BY 4.0. Data published by United Nations, Department of Economic and Social Affairs, Population Division (2019). World Population Prospects: The 2019 Revision, DVD edition. https://population.un.org/wpp2019/Download/Standard/Interpolated/.

in sub-Saharan Africa and South Asia. But we are making progress (Figure 1.6).

All these advances—declines in extreme poverty, undernourishment, and maternal and child mortality—reflect a world where the conditions that shape health have improved. In historical terms, this improvement has been remarkably sudden. Economic, scientific, political, and technological forces have created in the last two centuries standards of living that the majority of people who have ever existed on the earth could scarcely have imagined, much less hoped to experience themselves. Perhaps the most striking aspect of this achievement in health is that it was, for the most part, unintentional. When we think of human milestones, we often think of them coming about like this: we collectively set a goal—landing on the moon, say—then work toward it, succeeding only after years of focused effort. This makes it

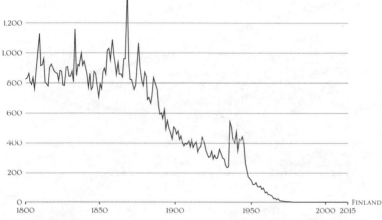

MATERNAL MORTALITY RATIO, 1800 TO 2015

THE MATERNAL MORTALITY RATIO IS THE NUMBER OF WOMEN WHO DIE FROM
PREGNANCY-RELATED CAUSES WHILE PREGNANT OR WITHIN 42 DAYS OF
PREGNANCY TERMINATION PER 100,000 LIVE BIRTHS.

Figure 1.5. Adapted from figure found at Roser M. Measurement Matters—The Decline of Maternal Mortality. Our World in Data website. https://ourworldindata.org/measurement-matters-the-decline-of-maternal-mortality. Published October 25, 2017. Accessed December 31, 2020. Licensed under CC BY 4.0. Historical data (up to 1979) Gapminder. Historical estimates reconstructed by Hanson C in 2010. The work is documented here: https://www.gapminder.org/documentation/documentation/gapdoc010.pdf. And accessible here: https://docs.google.com/spreadsheets/d/14ZtQy9kdopMRKWg_zKsTg3qKHoGtflj-Ekal9gIPZ4A/pub#. Recent data (1990 to 2015): WHO, UNICEF, UNFPA, World Bank Group, United Nations Population Division. *Trends in Maternal Mortality: 1990 to 2015*. Geneva: World Health Organization; 2015.

all the more significant that a key victory for humanity—raising life expectancy by creating the healthiest time in our history—was not the result of targeted effort toward the specific goal of health. Rather, it was a byproduct of foundational forces unfolding over time, forces including industrialization, global development, urbanization, and political changes. The better health this has wrought remains worth celebrating—success is success, regardless of whether or not we were aiming for it. However, the incidental nature of this success has meant

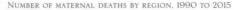

NUMBER OF MATERNAL DEATHS BY REGION, 1990 TO 2015

A MATERNAL DEATH REFERS TO THE DEATH OF A WOMAN WHILE PREGNANT OR WITHIN 42 DAYS
OF TERMINATION OF PREGNANCY, IRRESPECTIVE OF THE DURATION AND SITE OF THE PREGNANCY,
FROM ANY CAUSE RELATED TO OR AGGRAVATED BY THE PREGNANCY OR ITS MANAGEMENT BUT
NOT FROM ACCIDENTAL OR INCIDENTAL CAUSES.

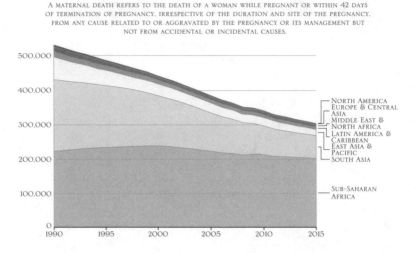

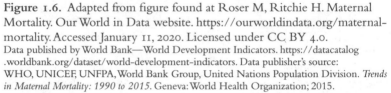

Figure 1.6. Adapted from figure found at Roser M, Ritchie H. Maternal Mortality. Our World in Data website. https://ourworldindata.org/maternal-mortality. Accessed January 11, 2020. Licensed under CC BY 4.0.
Data published by World Bank—World Development Indicators. https://datacatalog .worldbank.org/dataset/world-development-indicators. Data publisher's source: WHO, UNICEF, UNFPA, World Bank Group, United Nations Population Division. *Trends in Maternal Mortality: 1990 to 2015.* Geneva: World Health Organization; 2015.

that we have yet to fully acknowledge why it occurred, which hinders our ability to advance it in the future. Most of us still think of health as a product of medicine rather than as an emergent property of social, economic, environmental, and political forces. When we compare health in the present to health a century ago, we are still liable to attribute our gains to better medicine. As a result, we are in the curious position of having achieved something unprecedented while fundamentally misunderstanding how we did it. It is like landing humans on the moon without acknowledging the debt the voyage owed to rockets and physics. We have arrived at an extraordinary time for health with little awareness of the currents that carried us here.

Does this really matter? Is it not enough that we have arrived at a better and healthier time to be alive than ever before? Why do we need to know how we got here? The reasons are twofold. First, our understanding of the causes of health shapes our investment in health. In the United States, this investment is vast, far outstripping that of other countries (Figure 1.7).

We pour money into the pursuit of what we think will make us healthy. And what is it we think will make us healthy? Right now, the answer is overwhelmingly healthcare. The majority of the money we set aside for health goes to doctors, pharmaceuticals, and treatments. This has placed healthcare among the fastest-growing industries in the United States, with biotechnology and personalized medicine among its thriving subsectors. Now, there is nothing intrinsically wrong with such investment. These are necessary sectors, and it is right that we work to develop them. I am also in no way against doctors and medicines. I am a doctor, and should I become sick, I would want the best of my profession on hand, equipped with the best possible treatments,

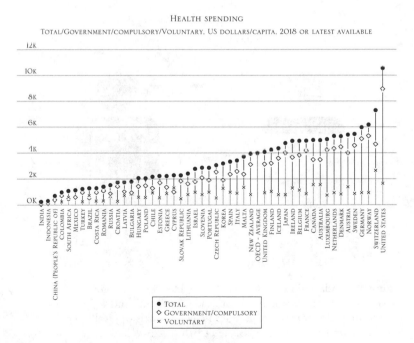

Figure 1.7. Adapted from figure found at Health Spending (Indicator). OECD Data website. https://data.oecd.org/healthres/health-spending.htm. Accessed January 11, 2020.

to help make me better. And I would want nothing less for anyone else. The trouble is when our investment in healthcare comes at the expense of our investment in the foundational drivers of health. It could well be argued that our investment in health should be reversed, and we should be spending more on addressing the forces that decide whether or not we get sick in the first place, rather than spending all our money on treatments for when disease has already taken hold. However, even those who do not accept this argument should be able to agree that our investment should at least be proportional, funding healthcare and health in equal measure. Our current investment is nowhere near proportional. While it is hard to precisely quantify the constituent pieces of what causes health, and even to precisely quantify how we spend our money (largely because there is quite a bit of overlap between categories), Figure 1.8 compares what shapes our health with where our health spending goes. It is not even close. On the left are the factors that influence our health, which emerge from the world

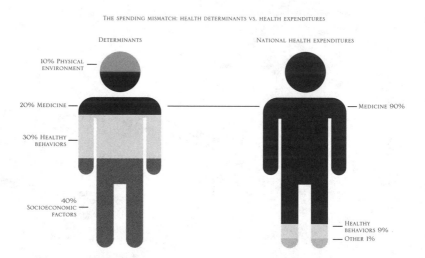

THE SPENDING MISMATCH: HEALTH DETERMINANTS VS. HEALTH EXPENDITURES

DETERMINANTS

NATIONAL HEALTH EXPENDITURES

10% PHYSICAL ENVIRONMENT

20% MEDICINE

30% HEALTHY BEHAVIORS

40% SOCIOECONOMIC FACTORS

MEDICINE 90%

HEALTHY BEHAVIORS 9%
OTHER 1%

Figure 1.8. Adapted from Healthy People/Healthy Economy: An Initiative to Make Massachusetts the National Leader in Health and Wellness. 2015. Data from NEHI 2013. Tarlov A. Social Determinants of Health: The Sociobiological Translation. In: Blane D, Brunner E, Wilkinson R (Editors). *Health and Social Organization: Towards a Health Policy for the 21st Century.* London: Routledge; 1996. Bostonfoundation.org.

around us—socioeconomic status, the physical environment, and the interaction of these health determinants. On the right is the $3.6 trillion we spent on medical services, at the expense of investing in the factors that actually determine health.

This misinvestment has meant that health in the United States has remained mediocre relative to that in comparable countries. This is not to say our health is bad. The United States is a wealthy country and has led the way on the advances in living standards we have been discussing. These advances have meant that the United States has much better health than many nations. But because we have not made a deliberate, targeted effort to invest in the foundational drivers of health, our health is far from where it needs to be. Yes, it has improved dramatically over the past century, but it lags far behind where it should be, and where it needed to be for us to be able to take Covid-19 in stride. That is why, for all our wealth, we were unprepared for Covid-19. And that is why we will be unprepared for the next contagion unless we change course.

This leads to the second reason it matters that we understand the true causes of health: if we do not, we will be unable to build a world that is ready for the next pandemic. Being prepared for a pandemic does not just mean having plans in place to deal with outbreaks when they occur. It means cultivating conditions that are supportive of health and hostile to the emergence and spread of disease. They are the same conditions that made the difference between the life of the child born in 1900 and the life of the child born in 1990. And they are at the heart of improvements in health around the world.

Let us return to one of these improvements—reductions in child mortality. Figure 1.9 shows the risk factors that contribute to deaths of children under five. None of these risk factors is more than tangentially linked to healthcare. All are shaped by the conditions in which children are born and live. Poor sanitation and unsafe water sources are linked to poverty, place, and community infrastructure. Air pollution is also linked to place, as well as to political choices that determine where residential spaces, roadways, and pollution-producing factories can be built.

If we neglect these conditions in favor of technology and treatments, we risk slowing or even reversing the progress we have made, and that means we are building our future on shaky ground. Child mortality has gone down because conditions have improved. But the

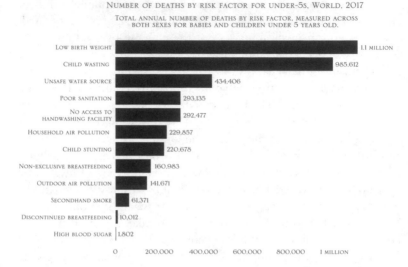

NUMBER OF DEATHS BY RISK FACTOR FOR UNDER-5S, WORLD, 2017

TOTAL ANNUAL NUMBER OF DEATHS BY RISK FACTOR, MEASURED ACROSS
BOTH SEXES FOR BABIES AND CHILDREN UNDER 5 YEARS OLD.

LOW BIRTH WEIGHT	1.1 MILLION
CHILD WASTING	985,612
UNSAFE WATER SOURCE	434,406
POOR SANITATION	293,135
NO ACCESS TO HANDWASHING FACILITY	292,477
HOUSEHOLD AIR POLLUTION	229,857
CHILD STUNTING	220,678
NON-EXCLUSIVE BREASTFEEDING	160,983
OUTDOOR AIR POLLUTION	141,671
SECONDHAND SMOKE	61,371
DISCONTINUED BREASTFEEDING	10,012
HIGH BLOOD SUGAR	1,802

0   200,000   400,000   600,000   800,000   1 MILLION

Figure 1.9. Adapted from figure found at Number of Deaths by Risk Factor for Under-5s, World, 2017. Our World in Data website. https://ourworldindata.org/grapher/deaths-by-risk-under5s. Accessed January 11, 2020. Licensed under CC BY 4.0. Data published by: Global Burden of Disease Collaborative Network. Global Burden of Disease Study 2017 (GBD 2017) Results. Seattle, United States: Institute for Health Metrics and Evaluation (IHME), 2018.

continued existence of child mortality shows how much work we have left to do to build a healthier world. The same could be said of all the markers of progress covered in this chapter. We have come far, but we are not where we should be, as the Covid-19 moment has shown.

But there is reason to be encouraged that the present could evolve into a radically healthier world if we chart the right course now. The fact that we have come so far over the last two centuries without having the goal of health explicitly in mind suggests that if we were to choose collectively to shape the conditions of our world with an eye toward health, the result could be transformative. Imagine what we could do if we designed our world with the central goal of improving health. If we invested more in the communities left behind by economic development, to help their boats reach the highest level. Or if we channeled our efforts at urban planning into creating cities that maximize the health of their inhabitants. We could make the present moment, with all its outstanding progress, merely the prelude to an even healthier future.

Covid-19 was perhaps the strongest case that could be made for taking these steps. The challenge of Covid-19 was not just in the emergence of a novel virus. The virus was clearly a problem, of course, and the core cause of the disruption we faced. But it only became what it became because it found us unprepared, lazily thinking our health was fine. We did not invest in health when times were good. So when times became not so good, we had to scramble to adjust, to cope—and not every adjustment the moment called for was feasible on such short notice.

Covid-19 has shown the need for a long-term plan for promoting health on a global scale. The last century saw the advance of broad improvements in standards of living, but the pace of progress masked the fact that these advances were largely rudderless. With the winds steering our ship toward a better day for health, we did not need to chart a course with any specificity. Now, however, it is necessary for us to take ownership of our voyage. The twenty-first century has shown how quickly the winds can change. We cannot rely on them to carry us to where we need to be when the next pandemic strikes. We need a clearly defined plan for the rest of the century and beyond if we wish to expand the gains we have already made and generate improvement in areas our progress has not yet fully reached.

If we can do this, the child born in 2100 could be far better off than the child born in 1990. What might life be like for this child? She would grow up with abundant access to the food, shelter, and education that support healthy development. Her access to such resources would be sustained by strategic investment in her community, the result of government initiatives aimed at promoting population health. We can imagine these initiatives being launched to counteract the effects of automation, helping newly unemployed populations thrive during a period of economic transition. These initiatives might include investment in green spaces, transportation infrastructure, and environmental protection, and they might also include putting cash directly in the hands of those who need it through the adoption of a universal basic income. Perhaps there will be some controversy over whether such spending is justified before policymakers ultimately act in accordance with the data linking such investment to better health. This decision could be motivated by an international resolution, adopted in the aftermath of Covid-19, for governments to measure the health impacts of all policies under consideration, in order to craft laws that support better health for all.

This approach to health could create a context where the child can live a life largely free from preventable disease. While the creation of this context, driven by political will and data-informed action, would be a historic achievement, the most significant aspect of the child's story would be her place of birth—which in that world could be any-where. Central to this vision of the future will be a focus on areas that did not fully share in the economic development of the nineteenth and twentieth centuries. This entails the international community deciding to create a world where a child can be born anywhere and enjoy equal access to the resources that enable health. So as the world applies its energy and commitment to building a better future, it prioritizes the areas where this effort is needed most.

It is entirely within our power to usher in a future like the one I have just described. Doing so means recognizing the forces that have already made our world healthier than it has ever been, and engag-ing with these forces to make the world even better. It also means acknowledging how these forces, when left to their own devices, can create inequalities, which we must make a conscious, concerted effort to address. Being healthy and prepared for the next pandemic requires us to first see all the ways we are still unhealthy, even in the midst of progress.

2

An Unhealthy Country

During the Covid-19 pandemic, Michael Hobbes wrote a piece in *HuffPost* titled "Will America Let COVID-19 Become the Next HIV?" The question was a good one. HIV is an example of how the divides within a society can allow a disease to flourish among marginalized communities while remaining far less prevalent among more advantaged populations. When HIV first entered our consciousness, it was primarily a challenge for men who have sex with men and for people who use intravenous drugs. While this was partly due to society's marginalization of these groups, the more salient issue was how the practices of these groups intersected with the virus's means of transmission. However, as we developed better prevention and treatment strategies for HIV, risk of the disease is now almost entirely mediated by socioeconomic factors. Current HIV drugs are of such quality that we have the capacity to drive the disease into statistical nonexistence. The reasons we have not yet met this goal are the economic factors preventing certain populations from accessing these drugs; the social stigma, which complicates how we address the disease; and governmental policies that, for political reasons, do not adequately address these barriers. So where we now find ourselves on HIV—in what are hopefully the disease's last years—in a sense mirrors where we were when we first encountered it in the 1980s, in that in both eras the burden of the disease fell most heavily on certain marginalized groups. The difference is that in the beginning, this disparity was largely a consequence of the nature of the disease, whereas now it is the result of socioeconomic divides we have allowed to remain in place. As we have succeeded in improving treatment, we have failed to address the structural causes of poor health, a mistake we continue to make.

Hobbes's point was that Covid-19 had the potential to follow a similar trajectory. From practically the moment it emerged in the United States, it began affecting some populations more than others, with the socioeconomically marginalized at greater risk. What is striking about this is that, unlike HIV, Covid-19 did not spread by exploiting the behaviors of specific groups; its method of transmission was closer to that of a conventional flu, making it more of a generalized threat than HIV ever was. Given this reality, the fact that its spread so quickly mapped onto existing health divides in the United States reflects the degree to which we have failed to address these divides, and reinforces the importance of doing so before the next outbreak.

During the past century and a half, health improved for so many that it is possible to believe that it improved at the same rate for everyone. But it did not. We saw these inequalities clearly during Covid-19, as racial, regional, and socioeconomic differences placed certain populations at greater risk of the disease. Such divides are deeply rooted and have long been with us. Among the starkest divides in the United States is the line between those at the top of the economic ladder and those at the bottom. I have already mentioned the nearly fourteen-year gap in life expectancy between these groups. The intersection of Americans' health and their economic circumstances is reflected in a number of other areas. Populations experiencing higher levels of economic disadvantage are also likelier to suffer from poor mental health and chronic disease. And they are less likely to have access to quality education, a deprivation associated with significant health risks of its own. Health divides in the United States unfold along racial and ethnic lines as well. African American men, for example, are likelier to die from prostate cancer than other racial groups. African American women are likelier to die from breast cancer. And Hispanic Americans are about 50 percent likelier to die from diabetes or liver disease than white Americans.

These same racial health divides characterized the spread of Covid-19 in the United States. Figure 2.1 shows Covid-19 deaths per 100,000 people among various racial groups through December 8, 2020, dramatically highlighting the significantly higher risk faced by the Black and Indigenous population.

These health divides reflect a core paradox of modernity—a world that is simultaneously far healthier than it has ever been and far less healthy than it could be. By bringing health inequalities to the surface,

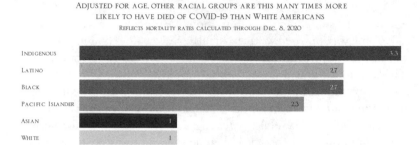

ADJUSTED FOR AGE, OTHER RACIAL GROUPS ARE THIS MANY TIMES MORE
LIKELY TO HAVE DIED OF COVID-19 THAN WHITE AMERICANS
REFLECTS MORTALITY RATES CALCULATED THROUGH DEC. 8, 2020

INDIGENOUS   3.3
LATINO   2.7
BLACK   2.7
PACIFIC ISLANDER   2.3
ASIAN   1
WHITE   1

Figure 2.1. Adapted from figure found at APM Research Lab Staff. The Color of Coronavirus: Covid-19 Deaths by Race and Ethnicity in the US. APM Research Lab website. https://www.apmresearchlab.org/covid/deaths-by-race. Accessed January 11, 2021.

Covid-19 complicated our narrative of progress. Again and again in the United States, we saw people sicken and die not just from the disease but from a status quo that significantly increased their chance of catching the contagion or developing a more serious case of it.

This unequal status quo emerged from the same forces that have shaped our country and our world—the economic, political, and cultural foundations of our society. At a perhaps even deeper level, in the United States it is informed by our national philosophy about individual freedom and the reality of how this freedom shapes our capacity to pursue happiness and health. This became particularly relevant on January 20, 1981, when Ronald Reagan delivered his first inaugural address as president of the United States, saying, "It is my intention to curb the size and influence of the federal establishment." His political rise had been aided by his ability to embody, to millions of Americans, the ethos of rugged individualism that has long been core to our national character. From the cowboys he played during his days as a film actor to the critiques of "big government" that formed the basis of his political career, Reagan was gifted at telling a story in which government bureaucracy curtailed the capacity of the individual to flourish, and all that was needed to reverse America's woes was a paring back of its administrative state. Operationalizing his philosophy while in office, he helped create a political consensus around disinvesting in the policies and institutions he believed hampered individual liberty.

Reagan's project continues to echo in the present day. It was embraced by subsequent administrations, Democratic and Republican alike, and was pursued with particular zeal by the Trump administration. It is a project with direct ramifications for American health. The agencies, regulations, and programs that constitute the "federal establishment" fulfill functions such as shoring up the social safety net, protecting our environment, and helping maintain a fair economy. Such functions are central to creating a favorable context for health. Disinvesting in them has steadily eroded the foundations of health in this country. It also left us vulnerable to Covid-19: it ensured that our health was already suboptimal when the pandemic struck, and it meant that we lacked the administrative capacity to coordinate our response to it at the federal level as effectively as we should have.

This legacy cannot be laid solely at the feet of one administration, of course. Our country's focus on individual liberty has also shaped how we collectively understand and invest in health. We believe health to be largely a product of lifestyle decisions made by individuals, and of the doctors and medical care these individuals are able to access. This has led us to overinvest in treatment and, often, to blame people for their poor health rather than look for its structural causes. After all, why look deeper for the reasons for poor health when it so clearly seems to be a matter of individual failings?

This has informed decades of neglecting the foundational forces that shape health in this country, giving rise to health gaps that prevented us from being as healthy as we could have been in the years leading up to Covid-19. At the same time, flaws and injustices in the country's socioeconomic system—some of which date back to the country's founding—have allowed particularly poor health to emerge among certain marginalized populations. This poor health, long minimized or ignored, did much to set the stage for our failures during Covid-19. This chapter will explore how the forces of foundational injustice and disinvestment in the structures that support health placed our health at risk during Covid-19 and continue to do so now.

The United States has the largest economy on earth. We have made spectacular gains in advancing social and political progress, moving in about 250 years from a slaveholding country where only white men could vote to a country where all enjoy equal political rights and protection before the law. These advances have intersected with overall rises in global living standards to significantly improve health in the

United States. Yet underneath this progress, there are still deep inequalities. Some are the natural inequalities inherent in a free economic and political system where, aspirationally, the only limits placed on an individual's ability to succeed are her own talents and abilities. However, some inequalities are the result of deliberate, targeted injustice, present at the founding of our social and political system, which has over the years excluded certain populations from the resources necessary for health.

Underlying all of this is our disinvestment in the core drivers of health, a misplacement of resources caused by our focus on doctors, pharmaceuticals, and treatments at the expense of engaging with the forces that truly shape health. Preparing for the next pandemic means first understanding the ways we are currently unhealthy in the United States, the deeper causes of this poor health, and how we can fix them. It means creating a country where no one faces greater risk of illness and death because of skin color, place of birth, economic status, or preexisting condition. Creating such a country requires us to take an honest look at how we have fallen short. We can do this first by looking at the following key metrics: life expectancy, addiction, mental health and suicide, and noncommunicable diseases.

Let us begin with life expectancy. In Chapter 1, comparing life expectancy across time helped illustrate the progress we have made in building a healthier world. The rise in life expectancy reflects improvements in the conditions that shape health. But life expectancy comparisons can also show how we are falling short. We know life expectancy in the United States is better than it was 150 years ago, and we know it is better in the United States than in countries where the resources that generate health remain hard for populations to access. But how does our life expectancy in the United States—and, by extension, our health—look compared with socioeconomically comparable countries? How do we measure up against our peers? In answering this question, we start to see cracks in the veneer of our progress. Figure 2.2 compares life expectancy in the United States to life expectancy in other economically comparable countries.

Compared with peer nations, the United States ranks at the bottom of the life expectancy list. The differences are not insignificant. Citizens of the country directly above the United States in this ranking, Germany, can expect roughly two more years of life than the

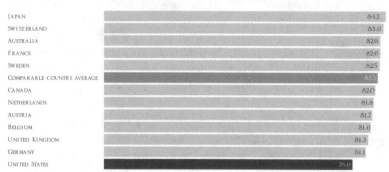

THE U.S. HAS THE LOWEST LIFE EXPECTANCY AT BIRTH AMONG COMPARABLE COUNTRIES
LIFE EXPECTANCY AT BIRTH IN YEARS, 2017

JAPAN	84.2
SWITZERLAND	83.6
AUSTRALIA	82.6
FRANCE	82.6
SWEDEN	82.5
COMPARABLE COUNTRY AVERAGE	82.3
CANADA	82.0
NETHERLANDS	81.8
AUSTRIA	81.7
BELGIUM	81.6
UNITED KINGDOM	81.3
GERMANY	81.1
UNITED STATES	78.6

Figure 2.2. Adapted from figure found at Kamal R. How Does US Life Expectancy Compare to Other Countries? Peterson-KFF Health System Tracker website. https://www.healthsystemtracker.org/chart-collection/ u-s-life-expectancy-compare-countries/#item-start. Published December 23, 2019. Accessed January 11, 2021. Licensed under CC BY-NC-ND 3.0 US. Figure data source: Kaiser Family Foundation analysis of OECD data. https://www.oecd-ilibrary.org/social-issues-migration-health/health-status/ indicator-group/english_bd12d298-en.

average American. Citizens of the country at the top of the list, Japan, can expect roughly five more years.

The life expectancy metric tells two stories. Seen over time, it shows we are in a better place than we have ever been. Seen in the moment, comparing the United States with peer countries, it shows our health is not yet where it could, and should, be. To make matters worse, in 2018 the National Center for Health Statistics reported that between 2016 and 2017 US life expectancy declined from 78.7 to 78.6 years. At the time, this marked the third consecutive year US life expectancy decreased. The last time the United States had seen such a decline was during the 1915–1918 period, which included deaths caused by World War I and the Spanish flu pandemic. It is significant that Covid-19 has been compared to the Spanish flu, yet the US experienced a decline in life expectancy before Covid-19 ever arrived on our shores, one driven by challenges such as suicide, addiction, and chronic disease. In a sense, then, Covid-19 was one outbreak among many, intersecting with a web of ongoing health challenges that created the context for a crisis of historic proportions.

Among the best-known of these epidemics is our national struggle with addiction, in particular opioids. Addiction-related mortality was a key driver of recent life expectancy declines, and it remains at the heart of our country's poor health. In 2018, for example, more than 67,300 people in the United States died from drug overdoses. As large as it is, this number represented a welcome decline in what had been up to that point a fairly steady rise in drug overdose deaths, from 38,329 in 2010 to 70,237 in 2017. Figure 2.3 is a visualization of this rise.

These deaths are largely driven by the use of opioids such as heroin and fentanyl (a synthetic, highly potent opioid), the proliferation of which is a product of many interlocking factors, including pharmaceutical marketing and prescribing practices, the illegal importation of fentanyl from China, and the increasing role of the internet in making the sale of illicit drugs easier. The opioid epidemic has also been sustained by the stigma our society still directs at people who struggle

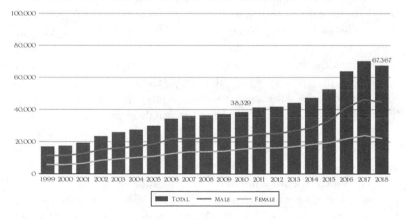

NATIONAL DRUG OVERDOSE DEATHS: NUMBER AMONG ALL AGES, BY GENDER, 1999–2018

Figure 2.3. Adapted from figure found at Overdose Death Rates. National Institute on Drug Abuse website. https://www.drugabuse.gov/drug-topics/trends-statistics/overdose-death-rates. Accessed January 2, 2021. Public domain. Figure data source: Centers for Disease Control and Prevention, National Center for Health Statistics. Multiple Cause of Death 1999–2018 on CDC WONDER Online Database, released January 2020.

with addiction. This has led to many people who should be receiving empathy and support being marginalized and shut out from the
resources they need to be well.

The confluence of corporate, cultural, economic, and political factors at the heart of this health crisis is broadly reflective of the same
confluence of forces that produces much of our country's health challenges. The stigma many people with addiction face is particularly significant. Stigma and marginalization, while perhaps less tangible than
the brute economic and political forces that are often the core drivers
of poor health, are nevertheless critical to the continued existence of
health gaps. They are what allow us to ignore the forces that make
us sick and postpone having the difficult conversations necessary to
improve conditions.

The marginalization of certain groups has meant not only that they
are less likely to be healthy but also that their lives are less likely to
be part of the public consciousness at all. Marginalization is not just
the political and economic act of excluding communities from the
resources they need to be healthy; it is also the psychological act of
applying an "out of sight, out of mind" approach to people whose
poor health we would rather not think about. We would rather not
think about it because it complicates the narrative of progress with
which we wish to align ourselves and because acknowledging this
poor health calls on us to do something about it. So the first step
toward making this country healthier is overcoming our bias toward
not seeing the ways in which it is sick. It is hearing the individual
stories behind the statistics that reflect health gaps. We need empathy.
Through empathy, we can transcend the privilege that often limits our
moral field of vision to see the very different lives lived by others.

Empathy means a willingness to look beyond our immediate circumstances. Indeed, none of the steps suggested by this book are possible without this core willingness. It is what allows us to see what is
not immediately obvious about health but which is nevertheless vital
to sustaining it. For many in the United States, it is possible to take
for granted the conditions necessary for health. We do not notice the
pockets of poor health among us, because we do not need to. We have
money and medications, we feel well represented in politics and in
the public conversation, and our family histories are those of gradual
socioeconomic improvement, not intergenerational hardship. One of
the best features of America is that this positive narrative is indeed the

story of many of the people who live here. But not all of us. Empathy can help us to see those who have fallen through the cracks.

Such empathy is particularly important when facing another driver of our country's poor health: our difficulty addressing mental health. Suicide is the tenth-leading cause of death in the United States. In 2018, 1.4 million people attempted suicide in this country, and 48,344 died by it. This reflects a significant rise in suicide deaths over the last decade, from a national average of 11.75 deaths per 100,000 individuals in 2009 to over 14 deaths per 100,000 individuals in 2018 (Figure 2.4). Among those who died by suicide, 90 percent had a diagnosable mental health condition at the time they died.

It is important to note that many of these deaths were linked to our country's political failure to adopt commonsense gun safety reform— in 2018, guns were linked with over 50 percent of total suicide deaths. They were also a consequence, in part, of our failure to treat mental health the same way we treat physical health. When our bodies suffer from injury or disease, we do not fear stigma when we seek treatment. Yet this stigma remains present when it comes to addressing mental health. This has hindered our ability to prevent not just suicide but the depression, anxiety, and lingering consequences of trauma that undermine the health of so many.

Stigma has helped obscure our country's struggles with mental health and addiction the same way that more overt forms of marginalization have made it harder to see other health gaps. Just as many of us would rather not see the reality of mental health struggles, we

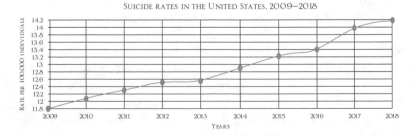

SUICIDE RATES IN THE UNITED STATES, 2009–2018

Figure 2.4. Adapted from figure found at Suicide Statistics. American Foundation for Suicide Prevention website. https://afsp.org/suicide-statistics/. Accessed January 2, 2021.

avoid seeing racism, poverty, economic inequality, and other factors that exclude Americans from health. This tendency toward avoidance suggests we are on some level conscious of these challenges, deeply so. Yet we continue to regard them as the product of weakness or moral failing, or else not our concern. Rejecting these attitudes is necessary for building a healthier country. Poor health is never a product of weakness, nor is it something for which individuals should be blamed or feel ashamed. The only blame that applies is the blame we collectively share for accepting the conditions that open the door to stigma and poor health in the first place.

The intersection of mental health and addiction reflects the core truth that the forces that challenge health are often linked. They overlap and inform each other, deepening their hold on our health. For example, mental health intersects with economic challenge, which can drive the distress that leads to suicide. The Covid-19 moment, with its consequences for the global economy coupled with the challenge of physical isolation and disruption of care, created what were in many ways the ideal conditions for poor mental health to emerge. The intersection of such challenges, then, creates the context for difficulties to emerge that are greater than the sum of their parts. The more hopeful side of this is that the conditions that promote health also intersect. This suggests that by working to improve health by improving these conditions, we can make the world not just healthier but exponentially so.

One area where this work is particularly necessary is that of noncommunicable chronic diseases (NCDs), which account for much of the burden of poor health in the United States. NCDs are conditions that cannot be physically spread from person to person (although we know that behaviors are also contagious, in a sense, and influence the spread of NCDs). Because they are not directly transmissible, NCDs tend not to generate the level of acute fear evoked by infectious threats such as Covid-19. Yet in terms of sheer numbers they have done far more damage to health in the United States than the recent pandemic. Hundreds of thousands of NCD-related deaths occur each year in the United States, accounting for 88 percent of all annual deaths in this country as of 2016 (Figure 2.5).

Pointing out how NCD mortality dwarfs Covid-19 deaths is not, of course, to try to minimize Covid-19 by comparison. The challenge of the pandemic and the challenge of NCDs in the United States are

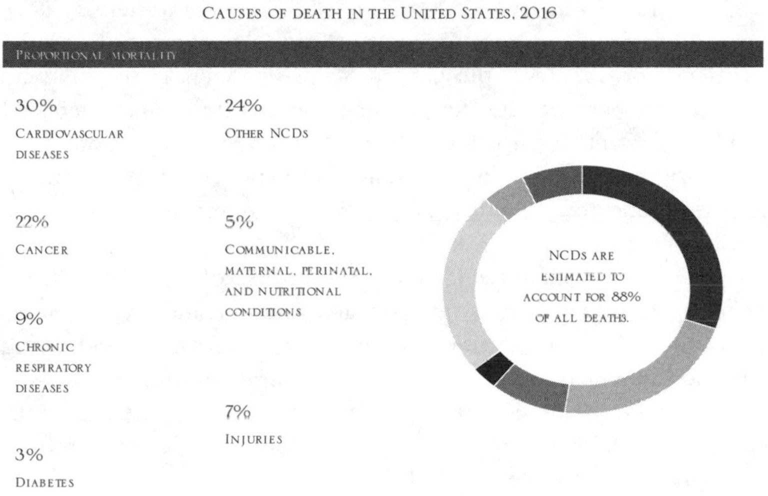

CAUSES OF DEATH IN THE UNITED STATES, 2016

PROPORTIONAL MORTALITY

30%
CARDIOVASCULAR
DISEASES

24%
OTHER NCDs

22%
CANCER

5%
COMMUNICABLE,
MATERNAL, PERINATAL,
AND NUTRITIONAL
CONDITIONS

9%
CHRONIC
RESPIRATORY
DISEASES

NCDs ARE
ESTIMATED TO
ACCOUNT FOR 88%
OF ALL DEATHS.

7%
INJURIES

3%
DIABETES

Figure 2.5. Adapted from figure found at World Health Organization. United States of America. In: World Health Organization— Noncommunicable Diseases (NCD) Country Profiles, 2018. https://www .who.int/nmh/countries/usa_en.pdf?ua=1. Accessed January 11, 2021.

closely linked. One of the first and clearest data points to emerge about Covid-19 was that populations with underlying conditions were at increased risk of complications and death from the disease. Chronic NCDs represent a high proportion of these underlying conditions, which include cardiovascular disease, cancer, and chronic respiratory disease. About 647,000 Americans die each year from heart disease. It is the leading cause of death in the United States, claiming a life every thirty-seven seconds. The challenge of heart disease is rivaled by that of cancer, the second-leading cause of death in the United States. In 2017, there were 1,701,315 new cases of cancer reported in this country, and 599,099 people died from the disease. The burden of respiratory disease is also substantial. Over 25 million Americans suffer from asthma—7.7 percent of the adult population and 8.4 percent of children. Since the 1980s, asthma has been increasing among all age, sex, and racial demographics. However, it remains more common among adult women than among adult men, and Black Americans die at a higher rate from asthma than other racial or ethnic groups.

Heart disease, cancer, and asthma are all linked to another signature American epidemic: obesity. From 1999–2000 through 2017–2018, the prevalence of obesity in the United States increased from 30.5 percent to 42.4 percent, and the prevalence of severe obesity increased from 4.7 percent to 9.2 percent. Given the range of conditions associated with obesity and its increasing prevalence, obesity is arguably the most dangerous health challenge facing Americans, even in the Covid-19 era.

In a sense, the obesity epidemic is the inverse of Covid-19. Where Covid-19 was an infectious threat that exploited underlying conditions, obesity is a noninfectious challenge that creates those underlying conditions—which can be exploited by any number of infectious diseases, not just Covid-19. Cancer, diabetes, and serious heart conditions were all among the factors placing populations at greater risk from Covid-19. When we see how vulnerability to Covid-19 links to these conditions, how these conditions link to obesity, and how obesity links to the larger forces that shape our health, we are faced with the unsettling fact that much of this morbidity and mortality was, and remains, preventable.

Why, then, do we not prevent it? To answer this, we must return to the issue of stigma and marginalization. When we think of the causes of obesity, more often than not we think of failures of individuals before we think of failures of systems. We often see obesity as the consequence of personal choices. There is a temptation to moralize about obesity, to attribute it to eating the wrong food and shunning exercise. This moralizing is not limited to how we see obesity. Our tendency to see health solely through the lens of individual decision-making can lead us to blame sick people for their own poor health, just as our Horatio Alger–inspired myths about personal initiative being the best corrective to poverty can lead us to blame people for their socioeconomic disadvantage. It is an easy outlook to adopt, but upon closer examination it does not hold up well. The causes of obesity are far more complex than a person's choices about food or exercise, just as the causes of poverty are far more complex than an individual's capacity to work hard. Obesity is shaped by culture, economics, corporate practices, and other structural forces that are out of the hands of the individual. Consider portion sizes in American restaurants, which have significantly increased in the last two decades—doubling, and in some cases tripling. Not only has this shaped how much food we eat in restaurants, but it has affected how much food we see as an acceptable serving in all settings, changing the culture around what we eat. And as widespread as the challenge of obesity has become, it, like most health challenges, does not affect us all equally. This is a particular issue for low-resource communities, whose neighborhoods are often "food deserts"—places where unhealthy fast food can be ubiquitous and more nutritious food harder to find.

Obesity, then, is a microcosm of how structural forces shape health conditions that, on the surface, can appear to be almost entirely a matter of individual choice and behavior. This contradicts our national narrative about health being largely a matter of personal choices. Our attachment to this narrative has prevented us from addressing challenges such as obesity at the level of fundamental causes. The lesson of obesity is that the poor health that leaves us vulnerable to pandemics is all the worse for being preventable, sustained as it is by a status quo we have chosen to accept. We are vulnerable to obesity because we have chosen to leave in place the structures that support this vulnerability. We have chosen to increase portion sizes; we have chosen to let low-income neighborhoods become places where fast food is easier to get than nutritious fare; we have chosen to blame the overweight when they experience poor health rather than turn that judgment on ourselves as a society. When I say "we have chosen," I am mindful that few of us make a conscious choice to keep these structures in place; more likely, most of us do not think about them at all. But not thinking of them is a kind of choice; it is tacit acceptance of a world that is not as healthy as it could be if we made the effort to make it so. This acceptance is, in many ways, more dangerous to our long-term health than acute disasters such as a pandemic because it leaves us open to the indefinite recurrence of worst-case health scenarios at such moments.

In this sense, the health inequalities that keep our country sick can be said to be truly tragic. In classic tragedy, a character is presented as in many ways an ideal individual, save for a single flaw—pride, say, or anger. This flaw is typically accompanied by a willful blindness on the part of the protagonist, a deliberate choice to not see the crack that threatens to make the ideal crumble. This blindness allows the crack to deepen and spread until it proves the undoing of the protagonist and, often, his or her community. We find ourselves in a similar situation in the United States. As a country, we have unparalleled wealth and power. Our resources have allowed us to create a society that is far healthier than it has been in the past. But we have a key flaw—the pockets of poor health that hold us back from being where we should be. These include ongoing epidemics such as obesity and addiction, and the health inequalities that have concentrated poor health among marginalized communities. As in classic tragedy, these flaws are compounded by our unwillingness to see them. Instead, we stigmatize individuals for their poor health, which allows us to ignore the structural causes of disease. In doing so, we have allowed these cracks to deepen and spread, so when Covid-19 arrived, it found a society already cut through with vulnerabilities.

Our refusal to see these flaws speaks to a truth about our country's poor health: it is a choice. The health inequalities that persist in our society have not been thrust upon us by outside forces. They are, for the most part, a consequence of conditions we have allowed to persist in this country. Covid-19 exploited these conditions. In this way, the challenges we may once have been able to believe were just the problems of a minority were actually a key factor in the threat we all faced from the pandemic. If we are to prevent the contagion next time, we must have a conversation about the ways the United States is still profoundly unhealthy, recognizing the pain that lingers beneath our progress. Such conversations can be uncomfortable. But unless we have them, our health will continue to risk shipwreck when the next storm approaches.

One of the reasons these conversations are uncomfortable is that they must necessarily draw a distinction between inequality and inequity. Both reflect conditions where some populations are not doing as well as others. However, inequality can exist in a society without reflecting a fundamental injustice, whereas inequity points to something more problematic than life's natural unfairness. When it comes to inequality, few would claim that all disparate outcomes are a consequence of injustice. It is true that poverty exists and has structural causes, but it is also true that some people make more money than others because of the level of hard work they apply to their careers relative to their peers. Some people have natural advantages in athletics, while others do not. Some people are born with a talent for the arts that others lack. These are examples of inequalities that do not reflect fundamental unfairness or injustice. A society that achieved perfect equality of opportunity would nevertheless continue to see such inequality of outcome. Far from being an injustice, this can be a boon to a society. It takes all kinds, after all, to make robust, thriving communities, with everyone contributing to the degree that they can, informing a rich diversity of skills and abilities. It is when individuals' skills and abilities are not enough, when structural injustices prevent equality of opportunity, that we see something distinct from inequality. We see inequity. Inequities are disparities in outcome that occur as a consequence of unfairness or injustice. The injustices that create inequity include racism, xenophobia, marginalization of LGBT populations, and economic systems that unfairly benefit the wealthy at the expense of the less well-off. When these injustices are present in a society, they can prevent equality of opportunity, so that no matter what choices an individual makes, she cannot access the success, security, or health enjoyed by more privileged populations. Inequity creates unnatural disadvantage among populations that ultimately holds all of society back, ensuring that the cracks in our foundations remain in place, threatening the integrity of the structures that support our health. Building a healthy country means identifying when inequality is, in fact, inequity, and addressing the injustices that limit how healthy a given population is able to be.

The presence of inequity is not unique to the United States, of course. Inequities occur across countries and cultures, creating structural barriers to health throughout the world. However, there is one area where inequity in the United States could be said to be uniquely American: the area of race. The United States is just 150 years removed from a system of slavery that shaped our culture, economy, politics, and even our geography in ways that are still deeply felt today. It is important to remember just how recent this history is, how there are people living today whose grandparents were slaves. Emphasizing the role of slavery in shaping health in the United States is not to say other countries are not also affected by legacies of racial injustice. But the historical immediacy of slavery's legacy in the United States, with its roots in this continent dating back four hundred years, to before the United States was even founded, represents an inheritance that is still very much a part of sustaining health inequities in this country.

The distinctly American quality of slavery's influence was captured in another inaugural address, Abraham Lincoln's second, where he named "American slavery" the cause of the Civil War and the root of the nation's difficulties. In singling out the specifically American nature of this injustice, he was not suggesting that other nations had not participated in the wrong of slavery throughout history, only that what the United States faced at that time was a distinct form of it, embedded as it was within cultural, economic, and political conditions unique to that time and place. The health inequities we face in the United States today, of course, do not approach the magnitude of the evil of slavery, however much they are informed by its legacy. They do reflect the particular characteristics of the American system, just as health inequities in other countries reflect structural characteristics in those places. They were not imposed on our society from above, but rather sprang from soil that we ourselves tended, and for which we bear ultimate responsibility.

For this reason, we all share some measure of blame for the fact that those who are Black in this country are likelier to be unhealthy than those who are white. While this disparity remains, the country cannot be fully healthy. And our present moment is, sadly, full of cases where it remains true. The infant mortality rate, for example, is twice as high for Black babies than for whites. Not only that, infant mortality is higher for educated, middle-class Blacks than for lower-class, less-educated whites (Figure 2.6).

During Covid-19, it soon became clear that Black populations were significantly likelier to suffer from the virus than whites. This was reflected by the data and by individual stories. For example, in April 2020, *Kaiser Health News* ran a story by Liz Szabo and Hannah Recht about a thirty-eight-year-old woman named Shalondra Rollins. In late March of that year, Rollins came down with a headache, then body aches, which her doctor initially thought were from the flu. By April, however, she was diagnosed with Covid-19. Just a few days after the diagnosis, she was dead.

Rollins's death was a tragedy for her friends, family, and community. It also reflected the ongoing tragedy of the country's poor health, further exposing the United States as a place where some people, through no fault of their own, are likelier than others to suffer from poor health. Because while Covid-19 was the key factor in the death of Shalondra Rollins, there were other factors at play that increased her likelihood of contracting the disease—and of dying from it. She was diabetic, worked a low-paying job, lived in Mississippi, and was Black. With the exception of being diabetic, none of these factors seem, at first, like they would have undue influence on health. All of them, however, reflect conditions that create unique health challenges in the United

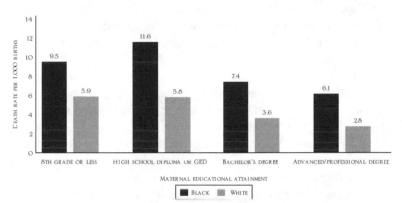

Figure 2.6. Adapted from figure found at Reeves RV, Matthew DB. 6 Charts Showing Race Gaps Within the American Middle Class. Brookings Institution website. https://www.brookings.edu/blog/social-mobility-memos/2016/10/21/6-charts-showing-race-gaps-within-the-american-middle-class/. Published October 21, 2016. Accessed January 3, 2021. Figure data source: Centers for Disease Control and Prevention (WONDER). Linked Birth/Infant Death Records, 2007–2013. https://wonder.cdc.gov/lbd.html.

States, placing health at risk in the best of times, and heightening risk during Covid-19. They are why Rollins could live in a country home to the best doctors and medical treatments in the world and still face an elevated risk of Covid-19. Working a low-paying job meant she lacked access to the resources that sustain health—not just medical treatments but the material goods that create a buffer against poor health. She was not alone in her disadvantage. The United States is a deeply unequal society, with increasing stratification of socioeconomic resources, exposing millions to the same disadvantage Rollins faced. This is particularly the case in Mississippi, where Rollins lived. As of this writing, Mississippi has one of the highest poverty rates in the country and the lowest median household income. This has created the conditions for widespread poor health, including chronic diseases such as diabetes, from which Rollins suffered. About 15 percent of the state's adult population has diabetes, creating a reservoir of poor health for Covid-19 to exploit. Finally, there was Rollins's race. As a

Black woman, she faced a disproportionate risk of poor health for all of the socioeconomic and historical reasons outlined in this chapter. The convergence of these forces made it unsurprising, though no less saddening, that Black populations were uniquely susceptible to Covid-19 in the United States.

Black/white health divides, from higher asthma rates among Black Americans to their lower average life expectancy compared with whites, are a uniquely American challenge, one that played an outsized role in shaping our vulnerability to Covid-19. These divides can be said to be uniquely American because of how they intersect with our country's fraught racial history. Being owned as property and then being subject to generations of Jim Crow laws and the denial of full social and political rights created for the Black community a level of disadvantage constituting a foundational flaw in the overall health of this country.

Systemic, structural inequity can ramify over time into a range of negative influences for health. These influences create a context where a healthy life is all but out of reach for certain populations. It is in this inequity that we see the complete picture of health and disease in this country. We can see how, in our era of progress, health inequities reflect something deeply against the grain of the better future to which we aspire. It is in no way natural that Black communities should be less healthy than white communities. It is the product of injustice sustained by a majority that feels like it has no stake in the challenges faced by the minority. Perhaps some feel a moral impulse to help alleviate these challenges, but how many do so because they feel that the poor health faced by the Black community threatens their own health and that of the entire country? This solidarity becomes possible only when we realize racial inequities are a problem not just for the communities who suffer from their direct effects but for us all. Because we are all implicated in the country's poor health, it is necessary to approach health as an extension of the common good. Health is bigger than any one individual, and it is ill-served when we dismantle the structures that support it—a trend enabled by our willingness to minimize the experience of marginalized populations such as communities of color.

In the context of our country's racial history and the poor health it has created, the death of George Floyd was all the more tragic, and the anger over it all the more understandable. The act itself was hor-rific enough; the implications of it, however, compounded its impact.

Occurring as it did as the disproportionate toll of Covid-19 on the Black community became known, the death of Floyd was widely understood to reflect the deep-rooted inequities that have undermined the health of the Black community in the United States. It reflected how we are still in many ways an unhealthy country. At the same time, the outpouring of support for addressing this inequity—including by having the difficult but necessary conversations about the history that informs it—suggested that the country was beginning to see how the poor health of marginalized communities threatens the health of everyone. The broad solidarity of the pandemic's early months, which saw communities come together in mutual support, developed a new focus as we saw that the vulnerability of communities of color exceeded that of white communities for very specific, very American reasons. Addressing these reasons became a key part of navigating the pandemic, and it remains a key imperative if we are to prevent the contagion next time.

If any good came from Covid-19, it was that the pandemic shattered the idea that the poor health faced by marginalized communities is merely the problem of those communities and that it is not fundamentally a product of the health inequities for which we all bear some responsibility. It is also worth noting that these inequities persist despite the steady progress we have made in the field of medicine. The fact that we remain so vulnerable to poor health despite this progress reflects that health really has little to do with the doctors and treatments we prize so highly and everything to do with structural conditions and our investment in improving them.

Becoming a healthier country means adopting a new approach, where we view the health of individuals as inseparable from the common good. This means looking beyond our focus on the individual and on the doctors and treatments that we have convinced ourselves our health chiefly depends on. When we see health as solely a matter of treatment and personal choices, we are liable to neglect the forces that truly shape health, to blame people when they get sick, and to disinvest in the structures that could keep us all well. We are also likelier to ignore the health inequities that emerge from our failure to see health as interconnected, with the health of the many dependent on the health of the marginalized few. This myopia about health also supports the attitudes of stigma, bigotry, and ignorance of history that can keep in place the structures that threaten the health of vulnerable groups in the United States. During Covid-19, these forces converged to make us sicker, but the time of the pandemic also contained the seeds of what it will take to make our country healthier—a new solidarity, concern for the common good, the beginning of an honest conversation about racial injustice and health, and greater prioritization of the political, economic, and administrative structures that support health.

3

An Unhealthy World

It is perhaps still too early to say if Covid-19 will prove to be the defining event of the early twenty-first century. What is certain is that the pandemic was this generation's first experience of an acute, large-scale trauma on par with the global catastrophes of the last hundred years. The twentieth century was a time when political and economic hardships affected millions on what was, in historical terms, a fairly regular basis. Two world wars, the revolutionary upheavals of the Soviet Union and China, the threat of nuclear annihilation during the Cold War—the advance of history in the last century was quite hazardous to the health and well-being of the global community. Modernity certainly brought progress, connecting millions through new technologies, uniting us in cities where more and more of us now lived, and bringing us together in worldwide social movements. But these developments were double-edged, carrying the potential for trauma on a massive scale in densely populated urban areas, a burden of civil unrest shared by the entire world, and the fear of global war that could end the human race.

Since roughly the end of the Cold War, it has been possible to believe that the world no longer faces the threat of such large-scale shocks. During the last thirty years, the world has seen neither global war, nor nuclear-tipped ideological conflict, nor the sacrifice of tens of millions in the name of political ideology. While many still live who experienced such challenges firsthand, the memory of global existential threats has largely faded. What threats remain have been largely localized. There have been wars, but they were regional conflicts, not global events. There were disease outbreaks—Ebola, for example—but they, too, were confined to specific localities. The world experienced troubles, but always in such a way that the majority of people could feel like these challenges were happening somewhere else, out of sight and, often, out of mind.

This arguably compounded the shock of Covid-19. When the pandemic struck, we were taken aback by the virus itself and by the sense that it was something completely new, all the more disruptive for being so unprecedented. While this impression may not have been accurate in historical terms, it was true within the limits of recent experience. This helped make the pandemic seem less like a reflection of the inevitable perils of life and more like a meteor striking out of nowhere, upending society as we know it. Had Covid-19 happened during the mid-twentieth century, with the global community perhaps better prepared to take such a challenge in stride, it might not have made such an impression on our collective psychology. After all, large outbreaks like the global flu of 1958 did not disrupt life anywhere near as much as the Covid-19 pandemic did. The Covid-19 era has seemed uniquely uncertain because of the sense of relative stability it disrupted.

I use the word "sense" here quite deliberately, because it is worth asking how accurate our impression of the pre-Covid-19 era was. Was that era really as free from widespread challenge as it seemed? Or was this impression to some extent illusory? Engaging with these questions is important not just for understanding what happened during Covid-19 but also for seeing clearly the forces that shape health in all eras. To create a healthier world, it is first necessary to be able to see the world as it really is, so that we can then take data-informed steps to improve it. An inaccurate view of the world—seeing it either as a place of steady and inevitable progress or as a place of irredeemable sickness and suffering—ill serves these efforts.

What, then, do the data tell us about the world as it was in the lead-up to Covid-19? As with the United States, where a century of progress masked deep health disparities, the global picture, seen through the lens of data, is one that is far from full health. It shows populations that were under stress from a range of challenges—from chronic disease to childhood mortality to communicable threats—long before Covid-19. Certainly, the world is healthier than it has been in the past. But the notion that Covid-19 struck a global population unused to large-scale health threats is simply false.

Why, then, were so many able to believe this fiction? The answer lies in the way the world is structured. Our present era is characterized by sharp divides between those who bear the burden of poor health and those who do not. Threats to population health, in their most acute form, have indeed become regional, deeply affecting some countries while troubling other countries less or not at all. These divides protect the healthiest not just from the effects of widespread sickness but, often, from even the knowledge of it. Those of us who are fortunate to live in the healthiest countries tend to be insulated from understanding just how much populations beyond our borders suffer, how poor health is endemic to certain places. In the United States, for example, the average American enjoys the expectation of being able to live into her seventies and eighties, with many of those years healthy ones. In other countries, however, the prevailing expectation is of a shorter, sicker life.

What shapes these divides? Fundamentally, much about them comes down to race and socioeconomic status. Chapter 2 addressed how these factors inform our myopia about health in the United States. These underlying conditions have created, in essence, multiple countries within a single national border, where some groups face radically different health outcomes than others based on factors out of their control. Because poor health is so often segregated—a word I use here quite deliberately—within certain communities, it is possible for many in the United States to live their entire lives without seeing how hard life can be for their fellow citizens. In this respect, the United States is a microcosm of the world. We live in a world where some receive the expectation of health as an inheritance—passed on to them by the favorable conditions into which they are born—while others are consigned by geography, race, or socioeconomic status to health being constantly out of reach.

Yet the fact that the burden of poor health is not shared by all does not mean it does not pose a threat to all. Covid-19 was a reminder that the health of all is interconnected: that health and disease in Wuhan, China, shape health and disease in Boston, Massachusetts; that the capacity of Europe to respond to a pandemic has implications for health in South America; that when one country fails to contain the spread of disease, it threatens the capacity of all countries to do so.

This principle of connectivity holds not just in times of pandemic but at all times. Although we may not often think about it, whenever

anyone anywhere is threatened by poor health, our own health is also
threatened, wherever we live. It does not matter how seemingly remote
this threat happens to be. We can only be healthy when everyone is
healthy. Being able to live in a healthy household, neighborhood, town,
or city depends on these places being in a healthy world. Covid-19 has
shown that disease does not respect borders. Promoting health at the
local level means promoting it at the global level.

Seen in this context, the world that faced Covid-19 was not a world
free of existential threats; it was merely free from the widespread
knowledge of them. As long as any part of our world remains vulnerable to poor health, we live, collectively, beneath a sword of Damocles;
Covid-19 was a reminder of the thinness of the thread that holds this
sword aloft. As the twentieth century was characterized by the threat
of mass conflict, the twenty-first is increasingly characterized by the
threat of mass contagion, driven by our modern connectivity and the
reservoirs of poor health we allow to exist. The shock of Covid-19 was
amplified by our willful ignorance of this risk. The pandemic revealed
just how vulnerable we have always been, and how vulnerable we will
remain unless we learn its lessons.

The first step to doing so is understanding the ways in which the
world is still unhealthy and the forces that enable this poor health.
As we saw in Chapter 2, this means, centrally, looking at health
disparities—the unequal distribution of health and disease. There is
much overlap between the forces that create these disparities within
countries and those that create them across countries. At core, health
disparities emerge from the misalignment of the structures that underlie health—the social, economic, political, and geographic factors that
unfold across time and distance to shape our world. Creating a healthy
world means engaging with health on this level—and we cannot prevent the next pandemic without creating a healthy world.

In this chapter, we will discuss how we can do so, first by looking
at the ways we have fallen short. The challenges of widespread disease,
the proliferation of unsafe behaviors such as smoking, and other forms
of preventable mortality all speak of a world that is still unhealthy. We
will then look at how these challenges intersected with Covid-19 to
shape health during the pandemic. Finally, we will look at the role
global cooperation and international institutions played in addressing
Covid-19, and their importance for creating a better future for health.

Perhaps the best way to understand how the world is unhealthy is by looking at an infectious disease that has in recent years killed millions and infected millions more: tuberculosis (TB). TB is among the top ten causes of death globally. Before Covid-19 struck, it was the leading cause of death from a single infectious agent. In 2018 alone, an estimated 10 million people were infected with the disease, and 1.5 million people died from it. Like Covid-19, TB is an airborne, infectious illness, which can spread through coughing, sneezing, and spitting. Also like Covid-19, TB is more dangerous to populations with underlying conditions, specifically weakened immune systems—making it particularly deadly to populations infected with HIV. Unlike Covid-19, however, TB is far from a novel threat. It has been with us for thousands of years, dating all the way back to prehistory. Yet we are fortunate that the history of TB has given way to a cure—antibiotics, administered regularly over the course of roughly half a year.

This, of course, raises a question: if we can cure TB, why does it still sicken and kill so many? The answer lies at the convergence of the structural forces that shape health. If ending TB were a matter of medicine alone, the disease would have long since been eradicated But medicine is just one of the factors that intersect with TB, and it is a relatively minor one. Far more important than the role of medicine is the role of poverty. Poverty creates the conditions of malnutrition, inadequate sanitation, and crowded slum living that help TB to spread. Poverty also undermines the creation of the robust health systems necessary for administering regular TB treatment. A core challenge of disease treatment and prevention is ensuring that once a drug is developed, those who need it can access it. This is difficult enough when the drug is a single pill. It is even more complex when the treatment is a six-month course of antibiotics that must be taken regularly. Administering this treatment in a context of poverty has long been an imperfect undertaking. The absence of strong health systems and the simple uncertainty of life on the socioeconomic margins can make it difficult to connect care with those who most need it. We saw a version of this challenge during Covid-19, when it was sometimes difficult to deliver effective testing to populations with low financial resources, populations less likely to have healthcare access. Such challenges can be even more pronounced in countries with significantly less resources and infrastructure than the United States.

Compounding the challenge of getting treatment to populations in need is the presence of stigma, which often accompanies the emergence of infectious disease. During Covid-19, cultural attitudes shaped perceptions of both the virus and the measures taken to address it, at times leading to stigma. Throughout the world, we saw how politically polarized attitudes, such as that against quarantining, created among some people a stigma against embracing measures that have been proven effective, to the detriment of health. That stigma can complicate the adoption of a health measure as seemingly straightforward as quarantining during a pandemic speaks to its power to disrupt the steps necessary for safeguarding health.

The confluence of socioeconomic factors including stigma and poverty has meant that TB has remained with us, despite our medical advances. It has also meant that the places where the burden of TB is heaviest are the regions most disadvantaged by the current distribution of global resources, notably Africa, where poverty, poor infrastructure, and an intersecting HIV crisis have kept levels of TB-related deaths high (Figure 3.1). Consistent with this, the growth of the disease has primarily affected the regions where it is already a significant challenge. In 2018, for example, 87 percent of new TB cases emerged in the thirty countries with the highest TB burdens. A full two-thirds of new cases were concentrated in just eight countries: China, the Philippines, Nigeria, South Africa, India, Indonesia, Pakistan, and Bangladesh.

The intense geographic concentration of TB in certain regions, and its near absence as a major threat in other parts of the world, has created a familiar status quo, in which certain populations experience a disproportionate burden of poor health. We have already touched on how this distribution of health and disease unfolds within the United States, shaping health disparities in this country. The example of TB is a striking picture of how this status quo shapes health at the global level. We can see the stark divide between those who suffer from acute poor health and those who do not. That TB is treatable makes this divide all the more an indictment of our willingness to tolerate the status quo. For populations privileged enough to take an "out of sight, out of mind" approach to global health disparities, Covid-19 showed us exactly what they—we—are really accepting in accepting this as the way of the world. The pandemic showed the world what it is like to fear an infectious disease that exploits socioeconomic conditions to undermine health, that threatens populations suffering from

DEATH RATE FROM TUBERCULOSIS, 2017
THE NUMBER OF DEATHS FROM TUBERCULOSIS PER 100,000 PEOPLE.

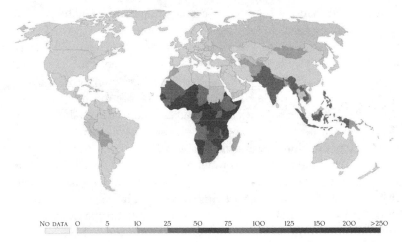

NO DATA   0   5   10   25   50   75   100 125 150 200 >250

Figure 3.1. Adapted from figure found at Death Rate from Tuberculosis, 2017. Our World in Data website. https://ourworldindata.org/grapher/ tuberculosis-death-rates. Accessed January 11, 2021. Licensed under CC BY 4.0. Figure data published by Global Burden of Disease Collaborative Network. Global Burden of Disease Study 2017 (GBD 2017) Results. Institute for Health Metrics and Evaluation. 2018. http://ghdx.healthdata .org/gbd-results-tool. Accessed January 11, 2021.

underlying conditions, that strains our health system, and that informs stigma that makes the disease much harder to address. We experienced this and thought it unprecedented, but the truth is that for the millions living in regions at disproportionate risk of diseases such as TB, daily life has long been like what the world faced during Covid-19—if not worse. The end of Covid-19 does not mean the end of acute infectious threats with the potential to undermine whole societies, just that they remain, for the moment, confined to the regions where they have long posed a challenge. The question we must ask ourselves is whether we will continue accepting this. If something like the Covid-19 crisis remains an indefinite emergency for some but not all, will we accept this status quo and call it a healthy world? Or will we realize that a healthy world is one where everyone is healthy, and demand of ourselves that we do better? If we truly want health, the answer can only be to restructure the world so that everyone can access the resources they need to be healthy.

It is worth pausing here to note that we are still near the start of this book and I have already suggested multiple times that the key to building a healthy world and preventing future pandemics is nothing less than restructuring the foundations of our society. Not only have I called for this multiple times, but—and here I should perhaps add a spoiler alert—I will do so many times more before this book is done. Why? Because this restructuring is fundamental to the goal of health. It is a necessary step, without which our health will always be mediocre, our populations always vulnerable to the threat of pandemics. However, it would be counterproductive not to acknowledge that this is also a very difficult task. Because it is difficult, it is understandable that some might mistake it for being impossible. It is a goal vulnerable to the criticism that it is mere utopianism, a castle in the sky that can only be built in the imagination. Such criticism might have had less weight in the context of Chapter 2, where the discussion was confined to the United States, but now we are talking about global health. A discussion of restructuring not just a country but the whole world is the natural place for criticism of the ambition I am calling for in our pursuit of health. Before continuing, it is important to meet this criticism directly.

So, is it indeed impossible to make the structural changes necessary for building a healthy world? Not only is it possible, but strategic decision-making that affects the foundations of health is actually quite common. It often occurs through the application of political or corporate power, or through the collective decision-making of international institutions. These actions are most effective when they engage with ongoing large-scale trends—such as population growth, urbanization, and the evolution of economic systems—that shape and reshape the world as part of their natural progress.

A key example of this is the growth of smoking in low- and middle-income countries. Tobacco use was once primarily a problem in wealthier countries. However, realization of its harmful effects sparked changes in the culture and economics of tobacco use in those countries, as tobacco companies faced backlash against their products and smoking went from being socially accepted to widely discouraged. This culture change, combined with laws restricting the sale and use of tobacco products, helped drive down smoking rates, notably in the

United States. This is perhaps the classic example of how engaging with social, political, and economic forces can indeed reshape societal structures to promote health. But it is not the end of the story. Faced with waning influence in wealthier countries, tobacco companies turned their attention to low- and middle-income parts of the world. Using marketing techniques honed over decades of dominance in higher-resource countries—notably, slickly packaged appeals to the young—the tobacco industry has sought to gain a foothold in these new markets. It is aided in this effort by population growth in these regions. These efforts have so far been quite successful, and this success has deep implications for health (Figure 3.2).

According to projections from the WHO, by 2030, 80 percent of global tobacco-related deaths will be in low- and middle-income countries. Many factors will likely be implicated in these deaths, from

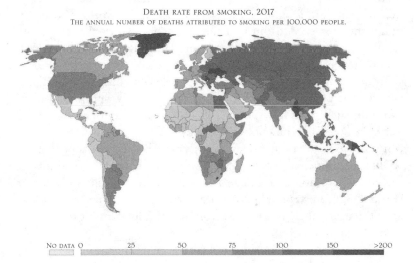

DEATH RATE FROM SMOKING, 2017
THE ANNUAL NUMBER OF DEATHS ATTRIBUTED TO SMOKING PER 100,000 PEOPLE.

NO DATA 0   25   50   75   100   150   >200

Figure 3.2. Adapted from figure found at Ritchie H, Roser M. Smoking. Our World in Data website. https://ourworldindata.org/smoking. Published May 2013. Updated November 2019. Accessed January 11, 2021. Licensed under CC BY 4.0. Figure data published by Global Burden of Disease Collaborative Network. Global Burden of Disease Study 2017 (GBD 2017) Results. Institute for Health Metrics and Evaluation. 2018. http://ghdx.healthdata.org/gbd-results-tool. Accessed January 11, 2021.

shifting cultural norms around tobacco use to the role of personal
responsibility in making the decision to smoke. Such factors are all
relevant, but the core force behind these deaths will have been a simple
choice made by a relatively small group of people. Tobacco companies looked at the emerging trends in certain regions, recalled their
earlier success in promoting their product through engagement with
culture and marketing, and made the choice to apply these insights
to the pursuit of profits in low- and middle-income countries. In
doing so, they embarked on a project that would affect the health of
millions. There is a tendency to think such consequential shifts can
only be the product of highly visible, clearly defined events of obvious
world-historical significance—wars and revolutions, for example, or a
pandemic. More often than not, however, they unfold more like the
global spread of tobacco—the product of quiet, commonplace decisions made by corporate or state actors with the power to implement
them. Such choices are key to determining whether or not we have a
healthy world. In looking at the ways in which the world is currently
unhealthy, it is easy to think of the long-term trends that shape the
status quo as entirely natural phenomena, even though they are, in fact,
deeply subject to human influence.

In the context of the global spread of tobacco, this may sound pes-
simistic, even slightly sinister. But it is really a fairly optimistic observation. It shows just how possible, even straightforward, changing the
world can be. Governments do it, businesses do it, and we, collectively,
can do it. It is not a question, then, of whether or not it is possible to
wield such influence. It is a question of whether we will wield it with
the goal of promoting health, of laying the foundations for a healthier
world. The more we see how we are currently falling far short of this
goal, the more likely it is that we will finally, fully commit to it in the
post-Covid-19 era.

The long-standing challenge of TB and the proliferation of smoking
reflect a world that has yet to make this commitment. We see this in
the 5.2 million children who died in 2019 before the age of five from
mostly preventable causes, in the 17.9 million people who die each
year of cardiovascular disease, and in the 9.5 million people who died
from cancer in 2018. This burden of disease and mortality is not something that simply happens to the world; it is something that emerges
from the world, from the foundations on which our societies are built.
Influencing the structural forces that shape the health of our world

requires us to first recognize how many of the health challenges we face are a product of conditions we have long accepted. The first chapter of this book is about how our health is in many ways much better than it has been at any earlier point in history. But better is not best. Getting to best means aspiring to build the healthiest possible world.

The Covid-19 pandemic created many examples of how the distance between better and best has made space for large-scale outbreaks to emerge. All of the health challenges I have mentioned intersected with the spread of the virus to worsen the pandemic's effects. Preexisting cardiovascular disease was found to worsen outcomes among Covid-19 patients and increase risk of death. Cancer patients with immune systems weakened by treatment also faced greater infection risk, to say nothing of the lockdown measures that complicated their ability to receive treatment. And the conditions that shape child mortality—poverty, poor sanitation, lack of access to nutritious foods, air pollution—are the same conditions that reinforce the health divides that did so much to help Covid-19 proliferate.

Consider, for example, the challenge of air pollution. It is a global challenge, killing approximately 7 million people worldwide annually. According to the WHO, nine out of ten people breathe air with high pollutant levels. The health consequences of air pollution include lung cancer, reduced lung function, respiratory infections, and asthma. The structures that shape air pollution include environmental regulations, the design of urban spaces, and corporate decisions about where to place factories and how to dispose of industrial waste. As with most health challenges subject to such conditions, the forces that drive air pollution risk also enforce disparities, so certain populations face a disproportionate burden of poor health. The design of cities, in particular, is a key factor in the distribution of this burden. Over 80 percent of urban residents living in regions that track air pollution face levels of pollutants exceeding WHO guidelines. Low- and middle-income countries face the highest level of exposure to air pollution; in the United States, this burden is often highest in nonwhite and low-income communities.

When Covid-19 emerged, the existing burden of poor health caused by air pollution helped amplify the virus's effects around the world. Air pollution caused by particulate matter was found to increase Covid-19 mortality in the regions where such pollution was present. Many of the chronic conditions that were found to worsen the effects of Covid-19 were conditions that can be caused by air pollution. It is, of course, not quite right to say air pollution caused these negative effects. What actually caused them was our choice not to comprehensively address the drivers of air pollution at the global level. We have long known that air pollution is bad for us—few realities are more self-evident. We have also made some progress in reducing air pollution around the world. That this threat still kills millions every year means our work is far from done. This calls for a new approach, guided by the lessons of Covid-19, to address the foundations of health in our world.

The role of foundational forces in laying the groundwork for sudden disaster is well illustrated by another disaster that occurred at the same time as the pandemic. In August 2020, lightning strikes caused a number of wildfires in the western United States, and soon these became record-breaking blazes, burning millions of acres in California, Oregon, and elsewhere in the region. The fires generated so much smoke that they actually turned the California skies red, making cities like San Francisco look like something out of a science fiction film. This unprecedented scene was caused by multiple factors. Lightning may have sparked the fires, but that spark became a blaze likely because of a combination of dry conditions, warm temperatures, a freak weather pattern that pushed dry winds toward the Pacific coast at a time of year when they generally do not blow in that direction, and state policies that did not sufficiently thin forests of the dead trees and brush that can help kindle wildfires. All this led to a historic disaster, which we struggled to mitigate as the fires raged seemingly out of control.

The comparison between the wildfires and the global spread of Covid-19 is clear. The virus was the lightning strike—a danger, a spark, but not yet a global conflagration. The burden of poor health—often heaviest in vulnerable communities—represents the weather conditions and kindling that allowed the spark to grow. In both cases, the conditions that acted as accelerants were sustained by a failure to create a safer, healthier context through smart policies and an understanding of the large-scale forces that, if left unchecked, increase the likelihood of disaster.

The conditions that created the wildfires also happened to intersect with what is perhaps the most significant threat to global health: climate change. I have mentioned the threat posed by climate change earlier in this book, and during the pandemic, I worked with colleagues to write an article for *JAMA: The Journal of the American Medical*

Association titled "Cascading Risks of COVID-19 Resurgence During an Active 2020 Atlantic Hurricane Season." The piece looked at the double threat that the year's hurricane season and the pandemic posed to vulnerable coastal states in the United States, to Puerto Rico, and to the US Virgin Islands. The succession of extreme weather events in recent years has bought attention to how the effects of climate change are unfolding throughout the world. The increased vulnerability of certain regions has shown how these effects disproportionately threaten certain populations—often populations that are already socioeconomically vulnerable, such as those in Puerto Rico who still live with the lingering trauma of 2017's Hurricane Maria. While some people in wealthier, more insulated countries—the United States, in particular—continue to debate the existence of climate change, the crisis has arrived for populations in these vulnerable areas. The threats of storms, droughts, wildfires, and displacement are a preview of what the rest of the world may face if we do not act on this issue. Doing so means addressing climate change the same way we should address other global health issues, such as TB—by addressing the foundational forces that drive these challenges. Climate change may not be a disease, but it emerges from the same conditions that influence the spread of disease around the world. Governmental policies, corporate decisions, economic trends, and changes in transportation and urban design are among the factors that shape climate change. The convergence of Covid-19 and hurricane season suggests how preventing the contagion next time intersects with the broader, generation-defining challenge of addressing climate change as a means of building a healthier, more sustainable world.

Addressing climate change is perhaps the quintessential example of why creating a healthy world takes global cooperation. No country can fully address climate change on its own, just as no country can unilaterally create a world that is protected against pandemics. Solving these problems takes nations acting together, guided by the goal of a healthier world.

Indispensable to this shared mission are international institutions such as the United Nations and the WHO. These institutions were formed in the aftermath of World War II, when the consequences of a lack of constructive global engagement were all too clear. Their purpose was to help coordinate global action in pursuit of the common good, guided by universal values. Perhaps the most significant articulation of these values was the Universal Declaration of Human Rights, proclaimed by the UN General Assembly in 1948. Among the rights enumerated was "the right to a standard of living adequate for . . . health and well-being." Health is indeed a universal value, and the desire for health is a powerful organizing principle to guide international action. The pandemic showed us that a concern for health can change how the world operates, as nations worked together to stop the virus. Such cooperation is a necessary tool for addressing the roots of poor health and creating a new global status quo in which we are no longer vulnerable to the threat of pandemics.

The decades since the founding of the UN and the WHO have been characterized by multilateral cooperation that has helped us to make progress on many of the core issues facing our world. However, this globalized paradigm has also created large groups who feel left behind by present-day economic and political currents. This has allowed a new nationalism to emerge, which prizes borders and cultural retrenchment over an open and robust engagement with the rest of the world. This political shift would play an important role in the years leading up to Covid-19 and in the world's efforts to address the virus when it emerged. Two core markers of this shift occurred in 2016: Britain's vote to leave the European Union, and the election to the US presidency of Donald Trump. Both of these events signaled a turning away from the international community toward a more contained, insular vision of nationhood. In each case, the arguments that a country ought to "go it alone" were accompanied by antipathy toward immigrants and countries viewed as competitors. The Brexit vote was, in part, a reaction to historically high levels of immigration to the United Kingdom, and the election of Trump was fueled by his denunciations of illegal immigration and his use of rhetoric that at times was xenophobic. The Trump administration, for its part, would go on to codify anti-immigrant and anti-internationalist attitudes at the policy level. It did so domestically through a more restrictive approach to immigration, and internationally through a more skeptical—even adversarial—approach to global organizations and agreements. Perhaps its most significant action in this area, in the years before Covid-19, was its decision to withdraw the United States from the Paris Climate Agreement. This move, a rejection of the global cooperation needed to address the climate crisis, foreshadowed Trump's later decision, during

Covid-19, to cut the country's ties with the WHO, claiming China had used the organization to "mislead the world" about the pandemic.

There is never a good time to cut ties with an organization dedicated to promoting global health, but to do so in the midst of a pandemic was—as many noted at the time—an act of historic recklessness. It was also a lesson—a clear example of how rejecting cooperation, rejecting internationalism, and rejecting working together as a global community toward the common good place health at risk. When countries turn their backs on the world they also turn their backs on the capacity to address the conditions that give rise to large-scale health challenges such as climate change and pandemics. And they hinder our ability to address these challenges when they inevitably emerge.

It is also worth noting that a nationalism that turns away from the world to fixate on its own borders can lead to the abuse of the people who wish to cross those divides. Often this begins as rhetorical abuse before becoming policies that directly harm the health of immigrants and would-be immigrants. We saw this in the United States, as Trump's rhetoric demonizing immigrants became a cruel policy of separating families at the US Mexico border. This dynamic is sadly familiar. Embracing division often leads to the groups on either side of the divide thinking less of each other and not recognizing their shared stake in building a healthier world, leading to dehumanization and cruelty.

Building a healthier world means choosing engagement over exclusion, acknowledging that just as the health of individuals is connected, so is the health of nations. When we think of our country as somehow set apart from the larger destiny of the world, we undermine our ability to make that destiny as healthy as it could be, while leaving everyone—our own country very much included—vulnerable to the consequences of this failure. This was the overwhelming message of the pandemic, but it was not received by everyone. The crisis motivated global cooperation, but it also exacerbated divides, which remain with us in the post-Covid-19 era. At this unsettled time, with global relationships evolving, power dynamics shifting, and basic tenets of the international order being questioned, it is important that the ties between countries do not fray, that we keep our attention on the common ground—our shared desire for health—that lets us focus on the challenges that affect us all.

Core to this task is understanding the long-term trends that are unfolding in the present era, so that we can leverage them into the creation of a healthier world. If the tobacco industry could use global population growth to its advantage, imagine what the global community could do if it chose to fully engage with the urbanization, global aging, and technological changes that are increasingly coming to define the twenty-first century.

For an example of what this could look like, let us return to the challenge of air pollution, a challenge that closely intersects with the ongoing trend of urbanization. Urbanization is a signature shift of our era. At present, over half of the world's population lives in cities. It's projected that in thirty years, over two-thirds of the global population will be living in cities—nearly 7 billion people. With so many urban residents currently living with poor air quality, the future of urbanization is central to addressing this defining health challenge. As new urban spaces emerge, we have a chance to shape cities with an eye toward promoting health. Imagine an international agreement on the design of cities—a commitment among nations to building healthier urban centers. These would be places that minimize pollution exposure, maximize green spaces, fully utilize transportation networks, encourage neighborhood-level investment, and promote climate-friendly energy consumption—all elements that help generate health.

Building a healthy world will take nothing less than this level of ambition. During Covid-19, we saw this at work in the push for a vaccine. The world acknowledged a common goal and the urgency with which it needed to be pursued, and worked together to achieve it, sharing data and leveraging the latest technologies. This is not to imply that the process was straightforward—on the contrary, working toward the vaccine was a complex task. Engaging with this complexity reflects the approach necessary for doing what must be done to shape a healthier world. The global health challenges that necessitate such an approach are no less urgent in the post-Covid-19 era. Climate change, pollution, infectious disease, and chronic disease pose an existential threat to health, ensuring that when the next pandemic strikes, it will be just as difficult to control as Covid-19, if not more so. In the meantime, these challenges keep the weight of poor health most squarely on the shoulders of the vulnerable. For much of the world, the pandemic was a moment in time—a difficult, dangerous moment, to be sure, but one with a beginning and an end. For the populations who suffer most from TB, climate change, and the many other challenges that keep our world unhealthy, the threat to health long preceded the pandemic and continues to this day. Their poor health is our poor health.

The experience of the pandemic caused the world to get together, to look for the medical technology we believed would stop the crisis. Preventing the next pandemic means understanding that the most effective way of stopping a contagion is not medical—it is structuring the world so that diseases no longer emerge. The place to start is where acute threats pose the greatest challenges, in the socioeconomically marginalized regions where Covid-19 was just the latest in a long line of such threats. In the early days of the pandemic, we all worked to limit transmission of the virus, through physical distancing measures meant to prevent an influx of Covid-19 patients from flooding healthcare systems. We did this with the understanding that the first step in addressing sickness is addressing where its threat is most severe. Creating a healthy world will take the same approach. By coming together to improve the health of the vulnerable, we can lay a foundation for the global collaboration that can bring about the changes we so urgently need. In the coming chapters, I shall talk a bit more about the forces that shape our world and our health, and how we need to engage with them explicitly to create a world that is resilient to contagions.

SECTION 2

The Conditions That Create Health

4

Who We Are: The Foundational Forces

The time of Covid-19 in the United States was marked by numbers, by the metrics we checked compulsively to track the course of the pandemic and take stock of the moment. There were the number of cases and the number of deaths. There were the number of immunization trials under way and the number of months until a vaccine would likely be viable. There were the shifting poll numbers, with their implications for the presidential election, a contest with profound implications for our national response to the pandemic.

Then there were the turkeys.

As fall 2020 began, *STAT News* published a piece by Andrew Joseph on the pandemic. Among the data and anecdotes that informed the piece was a vignette about Adams Turkey Farm in Westford, Vermont. The piece noted how the farm anticipated selling fewer of their "signature" Thanksgiving turkeys—weighing about twenty-four pounds—and more of their smaller birds that year. This seemed to reflect the reality of smaller Thanksgiving gatherings due to Covid-19. Judy Adams, the farm's owner, was quoted as saying, "We've weathered different things—certainly not a pandemic—but I just trust in the holiday, I trust in the turkeys."

This detail conveys an essential truth about the pandemic: it did not just strike our bodies, it struck our communities, our daily interactions, our livelihoods, our personal and collective foundations. The pandemic jolted large-scale political and economic forces, and it disrupted our most intimate shared occasions. It was the reason there were empty chairs around many a Thanksgiving table—or perhaps there was no table; perhaps Thanksgiving, like so much else, was conducted via screen. Because of Covid-19, our most cherished traditions—holidays, simple time with friends and family, big life events such as weddings—had to be postponed or else reimagined into something that fit within the framework of the "new normal" we quickly learned to adopt.

In the early days of the pandemic, it was as if someone had thrown a boulder into a swimming pool. The sudden fear, the mass lockdown, and the political and economic disruption came all at once, instantly disrupting our lives in big, noticeable ways. In the months that followed, the influence of the pandemic became subtler, like ripples extending in water. Life settled into new configurations, shaped by the presence of the virus. Homes, workplaces, recreational spaces, and the geography of communities were redesigned to meet the requirements of social distancing. Technologies were developed to allow us to live a more remote lifestyle, and to help with battling the disease itself, testing and tracing the contacts of the infected. As the pandemic progressed further, it started to become part of our culture. It influenced music and the visual arts, even the fashion industry, as clothing companies started making designer masks. It became a topic of daily conversation, shaping our political perspectives, the jokes we told, the hopes and fears we expressed.

Accompanying this was a return to a more fundamental way of thinking about the world and about the future. As soon as it became clear that the virus was to a great extent in control of our lives and would remain so for some time, we found ourselves in the position of having to live with a level of uncertainty that was, for many, a new experience. Because we simply did not know what the next day, week, and month would hold, and because we had so recently seen how quickly everything could be upended, we could no longer plan the way we used to. Plans became provisional; life became more and more about the contents of the day, about the immediate future, about what we might face from one moment to the next. The way we began thinking about the future was much like the way agricultural societies have long thought about what is to come. The farmer thinks in terms of seasons and the health of the next crop: "Will my fields flourish or lie fallow?" "Will the seasons permit a rich harvest, or will unexpected frost or blight ruin my prospects for next year?" The farmer does all she can to mitigate risk, but with an understanding that the future is fundamentally out of her control, that it will ultimately be decided by large-scale forces she cannot influence.

Covid-19 caused us to once again think like the farmer contemplating her crop. During the contagion, we did our best to plan, but we were forced back into the understanding that our lives are subject to contingency, that the future can only be viewed through a glass darkly, and that the deciding factor shaping our fortunes will always be foundational forces. These forces, as the preceding chapters have shown, are social, economic, environmental, and political. The dilemma faced by turkey farmers in the lead-up to Thanksgiving 2020 captures how the virus converged with these forces to shape a unique moment in history. The pandemic caused a lockdown that disrupted our lives to the point where safety seemed to necessitate staying apart even on important, family-oriented holidays. By allowing families to connect via screens, our computers created a middle ground between total isolation and taking undue risks to see each other during the holidays. Without this technology, tables might well have been empty and the holiday effectively cancelled, or they might have been fuller as the experience of unmitigated isolation caused families to decide that connection was worth the risk. The sale of smaller turkeys reflected the widespread settling of this new middle ground, as the culture shifted to a place it had never before been. Accompanying this shift were the economic consequences of such a move, as a more subdued Thanksgiving likely meant less revenue for turkey farmers—one of many examples of how the experience of Covid-19 reshuffled the economy, hurting some industries, helping others, creating uncertainty for all.

Perhaps the clearest example of the link between Covid-19 and foundational forces was the economic effect of the pandemic. From the earliest days of the virus and subsequent lockdown, it became evident that we faced deep economic uncertainty and potential crisis. In May 2020, data revealed that more than 38 million Americans had filed unemployment claims since March of that year. The economic writing was on the wall, and US political leadership acted by passing, with bipartisan support, a $2 trillion economic relief plan. A notable feature of the plan was its function of sending direct relief to individuals, in the form of assistance payments. This relief called to mind the ongoing conversation in some political circles about the possibility of providing such payments on a more permanent basis, in the form of a universal basic income. This idea had long been gaining traction as a means of offsetting the economic displacement caused by automation and growing income and wealth inequality. It had also enjoyed a recent boost in visibility as a central plank of the platform advocated by Andrew Yang during his run for the Democratic presidential nomination. Even so, the notion was still regarded by many as beyond the realm of political possibility. So it was striking to see lawmakers from both of America's major parties pass, with uncommon speed, a plan that included, if not permanent monthly payments, then something that at least reflected the spirit of the idea—no-strings-attached cash assistance provided with the understanding that material resources are central to supporting health.

In a sense, the economic relief plan was a clear-cut example of desperate times calling for desperate measures. Lawmakers who might generally disapprove of such government spending, particularly spending on direct cash transfers, would have perhaps justified their support for the plan along these lines, saying it was a necessary response to a crisis. Underlying this motivation is a central truth about crises: they reveal what is most important. In less challenging times, it is easier to take purely ideological positions motivated by theoretical notions about what is most critical to a country and its health, but when emergencies arrive, theory and rigid dogma are of little use. There is a quote attributed to Milton Friedman: "We are all Keynesians now." It suggests that even conservatives committed in principle to lower levels of government spending will, in a crisis, embrace the kind of outcomes-oriented stimulus advocated by John Maynard Keynes, because such spending has proven an effective means of lifting a country out of an economic hole. We reach for this tool because it works—it is as simple as that. Covid-19, too, fulfilled this function of turning us toward what we know works. We acted with the understanding that supporting the country during an unprecedented health crisis meant supporting the economic foundations of health.

Unfortunately, this moment of collective clarity about how federal spending can support health was the exception rather than the rule. Despite the fact that we cannot live healthy lives when we lack basic necessities, and despite the fact that our access to these resources is shaped by macroeconomic trends and the governmental policies that influence them, we do not always look at health through the lens of economic forces. It took a crisis like Covid-19 to reveal that these forces are, in fact, foundational to health, and that we cannot build a healthier world without supporting populations facing economic instability. The challenge is whether we will maintain our investment in the economic foundations of health in a post-Covid-19 world or decide once desperate times seem to have passed that we can dispense with the measures we took to address them. I say once these times *seem* to have passed because economic hardship will continue to create health challenges for large segments of the population, helping to generate the kind of chronic disease that amplifies risk during a pandemic, even after the Covid-19 moment has passed.

Consider, for example, how populations suffering from cardiovascular disease faced increased vulnerability to Covid-19. Around the time of the pandemic, I led a research team studying the link between cardiovascular disease and income level in the United States. We found significant differences in cardiovascular disease prevalence between low- and high-income groups, with a lower cardiovascular disease rate among the richest 20 percent. We also found this disparity increased in the years covered in the study (1999–2016). This study speaks to the central role of income/wealth in shaping disease risk, and to the broader message of how our health is shaped by underlying economic conditions. Fundamentally, it means that without economic interventions, we will be unable to reduce the pool of preexisting conditions that help opportunistic infections such as Covid-19 to spread.

It is worth noting that while the economic relief plan passed during Covid-19 was a clear effort to address the intersection of economics and health, it was not passed as an explicit public health measure. It was passed as what it most obviously was: a lifeline to businesses and individuals struggling in the face of unemployment and economic uncertainty. What is important to remember, however, is that when we are talking about unemployment and economic uncertainty, *we are talking about health*. We are talking about the mental strain that comes with being a missed paycheck away from disaster. We are talking about being unable to pay for the food that keeps us healthy. We are talking about being unable to afford the homes that give us security and shelter. Intervening to prevent such negative outcomes is intervening to prevent poor health, even when we do not realize it.

This is always true. It was true a decade ago, when we had never heard of Covid-19, and it is true now. The pandemic elevated the visibility of this truth while showing, perhaps for the first time, how dependent we all are on the foundations that shape our health. It may have been possible in, say, 2019 to feel sorry for those who were sick due to lack of the resources that generate a healthy life but to ultimately feel this was their problem, one that did not affect us directly. But the pandemic showed us how our health is intertwined, that my risk of getting the coronavirus was higher if more of us had the disease. This led us to see that the foundational forces that shape the health of some are, in fact, forces that shape health for all of us. And, as a corollary, we came to realize that when we do not intervene, when we allow populations to fend for themselves amid uncertainty, we undermine our collective resilience in the face of disease. Foundational forces are foundational in a very real sense. Like the foundations of a house, they are the bedrock on which we rest our society, our livelihoods, our health. Foundations, more than any other part of a structure, must be strong. If they are not, the house will always be at risk of collapse. It may not seem so; a house with weak foundations may go a long time appearing steadier than it is. But when the stormy winds blow, it will soon be obvious that what looked like levels supported by a strong foundation were merely floors stacked on top of each other with no proper grounding, upright yet precarious. This is why it is necessary, as a first principle for health, that we shore up the foundations on which our house rests. Health gaps driven by factors such as economic inequality are best under-stood as cracks in our foundations. Fixing these cracks, closing these gaps, means first acknowledging that they exist and are caused by our own shortcomings, then addressing them through smart policies and targeted investment. It also means not waiting until the crisis comes to think about the state of our foundations. Their soundness should be built into them long before they are put to the test, not hastily rein-forced when an emergency is already under way.

This will take a new way of approaching health. The work of addressing the economic roots of health is as much the work of chang-ing our thinking as it is about adopting the right policies. If a crisis can make us all Keynesians, the imperative of addressing the ongoing challenge of poor health can motivate sustained spending at a level typically reserved for historically unique moments such as Covid-19. Having seen the power of health to motivate bipartisan investment in improving economic conditions, we should extend the emergency measures of the pandemic into a durable commitment to reducing health inequalities through the use of data-informed federal spending. The pandemic made obvious why such an approach is necessary in a crisis; the next step is understanding why it is necessary for preventing emergencies, not just mitigating them in the moment.

Just as the pandemic shed light on the economic foundations of health, the time of Covid-19 was inextricably tied to a shift in our understanding of the foundational force of race in the United States. This began with the data showing Black communities were more vulnerable to Covid-19 than white communities, but it was the killing of George Floyd, and subsequent incidents of police violence against Black Americans, that truly sparked a society-wide shift in our approach to this issue. The scale of the protests against police brutality, which evolved into protests against the broader challenge of systemic racism, was more than an expression of polite concern or a recognition of the increased visibility of incidents of racial injustice. Far beyond this, they reflected a real change in consciousness around these issues. Americans, in larger numbers than ever before, realized the deep injustice that had long been foundational to life in the United States. This realization prompted an outpouring of solidarity between those who have been historically marginalized due to the color of their skin and those whose privilege has helped insulate them from these challenges.

This realization was not shared by everybody. The protests faced criticism, as did the critique of American society they advanced. The link between racism and poor health was not immediately clear to all Americans, and some wondered at the urgency with which the cause was being pursued in the midst of the emergency of the pandemic. The power of the protests was in their demand that we see what is not obvious to all, and in their insistence that we sustain this focus until we have enacted the structural changes necessary for a healthier, more just society. This means making it clear why race is foundational to health, and why racial injustice makes us sicker.

Racism has been core to the country's poor health since its earliest days. This includes both systemic racism—namely, the legacy of slavery as embedded within present-day institutions—and the experience of racism on an interpersonal level. There are ample data on how the lived experience of discrimination contributes to poor health outcomes among communities of color. There is a long-standing link between the experience of racism and poor health, particularly poor mental health. In the area of physical health, we are continually learning more about how racism affects the bodies of those who experience it. For example, a 2007 study, "Racial Discrimination and Breast Cancer Incidence in US Black Women: The Black Women's Health Study," suggests that the perceived experience of racism may be linked to increased incidence of breast cancer among Black women. These poor health outcomes did not emerge suddenly, in the manner of Covid-19; they emerged over the course of centuries, as the direct violence of slavery became the denial of justice and resources codified by Jim Crow, which echoes in the present day in the legacy of generations of segregation and economic and political disenfranchisement.

The intersection of these challenges and the degree to which Covid-19 posed a greater risk to Black communities than to white ones reflect the urgency of addressing racism in this country. When racism is seen through the lens of history, and in the context of the many challenges it poses for health, it would not be too much to say that it has posed an even greater, more foundational threat to health in the United States than Covid-19. Indeed, seen from this perspective, this conclusion is fairly self-evident. Yet, with some historical exceptions, we have not addressed racism with the same focus we apply to acute threats such as Covid-19. We stopped the world for a pandemic. But when it came to addressing racism, more often than not we dragged our feet.

Why? It is not that racism was less of an emergency than Covid-19; it's just that at the time of the protests, Covid-19 had been an emergency only for several months, while racism had been an emergency for centuries. It had become so interwoven with the fabric of American life that it was possible for some to not even notice it. This was particularly true in the context of a novel virus that had suddenly sparked such justifiable concern around the world. Faced with this new threat, one need not have been unsympathetic to the cause of addressing racism to not understand why so many would march in the midst of a pandemic, setting aside the requirements of the lockdown for the sake of this—or any—cause.

This lack of understanding speaks to a core truth about how we think about the foundational forces that shape our health: we tend not to. Just as many of us do not think about the poor health suffered by marginalized populations, we rarely think about the forces that shape our own health. There are two key reasons for this. The first is that while we do not spend much time thinking about these forces, we do spend a lot of time thinking about medicine, because we assume that is what's most important to our health. With this thinking comes investment—we spend overwhelmingly on medical care without making a commensurate investment in the foundational drivers of health. It is worth returning here, I think, to the visualization from Chapter 1, comparing what we spend our money on to what actually determines our health.

It is not hard to see why our health thinking and spending are so skewed toward medicine. Medicine is, for many, a first encounter with the idea of health. We base a lifetime of engagement with the healthcare system on a seemingly simple equation, learned in the days when our physician was still giving us lollipops after each appointment: when we feel sick, we go to the doctor, and she makes us better. At first glance, this notion of health seems comprehensive, covering the path from sickness to a return to health, and identifying medicine as the clear mediator between these states. Yet it has a blind spot. It does not account for the factors that make going to the doctor necessary— the factors that decide whether or not we get sick in the first place. This blind spot exists for the same reason some were unable to see why the protests against racism were addressing a problem every bit as urgent as Covid-19: because the foundational factors that influence health the most are so ubiquitous, so close to the skin, that we are able to overlook them for the same reason we can overlook the nose on our face or the air we breathe. What is more, the nature of their influence is complex, the opposite of the simple "disease plus medicine equals health" equation in which we put so much stock.

Consider the area of mental health during Covid-19. At the time of the pandemic, I led a research team that studied the prevalence of depression symptoms among US adults before and during Covid-19. We found that the prevalence of these symptoms in the United States more than tripled during the pandemic. We also found a link between higher depression risk and making less money, having less than $5,000 in savings, and being exposed to a greater number of stressors. On its own, any one of these factors might not have been enough to tip someone into depression. But imagine a woman—call her Maria—doing her best to make it through the pandemic. Like the rest of us, she experienced daily anxiety over catching the disease, or a friend or family member being infected. Now imagine, in addition to this baseline stressor, that she is an essential worker and faced the additional exposure risk that comes with having a job for which she is not able to telecommute. Then add that she has less than $1,000 in savings, so had she lost her job during the pandemic she would have had little means to support herself and her two children, to whom she is a single mother. Now imagine that she suffers from chronic asthma, had not seen her parents for months during Covid-19, and lost one of her oldest friends to the virus. Few could experience such hardships without running the risk of mental health challenges. And it was far from just a few who faced such realities during the pandemic. Millions across the United States, and billions around the world, faced an unprecedented confluence of stressors that placed both their mental and physical health at risk.

This confluence was driven by the intersection of the pandemic with preexisting conditions within society that compounded the challenge of the moment. In our study, we saw this in the finding that while depression risk increased for all groups during the pandemic, demographic categories that were particularly susceptible to this risk before the crisis remained at greater risk during Covid-19. For example, before the pandemic, women faced greater depression risk than men, which remained true as Covid-19 unfolded (the reason for this disparity is itself a combination of foundational factors, best seen through the lens of our shared context in which women and men still face very different experiences of the world on account of sex/gender).

When presented in the context of one individual's story, the factors that contribute to depression risk can seem entirely personal, unconnected to the larger forces that shape our world. This impression is inaccurate. Maria's income is shaped by the economic opportunities she is able to access, which are, in turn, shaped by governmental policies and broader economic trends. Her asthma is likely a product of where she grew up and its proximity to pollution-emitting factories and transportation networks. Her fear of the pandemic is also a product of foundational forces—specifically, of our collective failure to engage with these forces in a way that might have prevented the worst of Covid-19, a failure we must correct in order to prevent the contagion next time.

And, critically, none of Maria's problems would have been solved by medicine alone. Even in the best-case scenario, where she makes it through the pandemic without catching Covid-19 or seeing it infect more of her friends and family, she remains in a precarious place. She still has little money, two kids to support on her own, chronic asthma, and, on top of all this, the added trauma of having spent months fearing the effects of Covid-19.

There is no pill for fixing this level of disadvantage. There is only our willingness to engage with the complexity that is foundational to health, working at the local, national, and global levels to shape a context that sustains well-being. A healthier world, a world resistant to pandemics, must be a world that prevents disease. A positive outcome for Maria would have been one where she could access the necessary services—such as counseling, delivered remotely during the pandemic—to help her through her mental health challenges. An even better outcome would have been for her to never have been vulnerable to these challenges to begin with. What would it have taken to get Maria to this outcome? It would have taken addressing the lack of economic opportunity that contributed to her minimal savings. It would have taken providing childcare and other supports to help stabilize her life as a single parent. It would have taken policies that address why many in the neighborhood where she grew up developed asthma—a complex task in itself, given the many factors that contribute to asthma risk. If this all sounds difficult, that is because it is. It would be easy to look at what is called for in creating a healthier world and decide that it is far simpler to continue pouring money into doctors and medicine than it is to address the foundations of health.

This impression is reinforced by a mismatch, often amplified by the media, between what we think poses the greatest threat to our health and what actually does place us at greatest risk. Figure 4.1 is a visualization of thirteen causes of death in the United States and the amount of media coverage these causes receive. Suicide, homicide, and terrorism are significantly overrepresented, while chronic diseases such as kidney and heart disease, which together affect hundreds of thousands of Americans each year and which are deeply shaped by foundational forces, receive substantially less attention.

It has long been the case that the media conversation has not always accurately reflected the foundational factors that truly shape health. During Covid-19, we were able to see this dynamic at work in real time. It was striking how difficult it was, at any given moment, to get a clear picture of how the pandemic was unfolding. The media's view of the crisis was constantly changing, shaped by new data, yes, but also by notes of alarmism, the pursuit of the novel over tried-and-true approaches to health, and politically tinged outbreaks of misinformation, amplified by the partisan context of an election year. This messy cacophony was a heightened version of what our conversation about

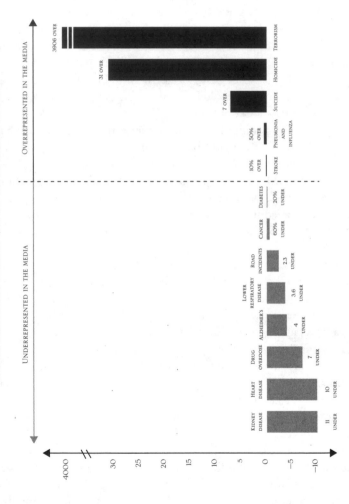

Figure 4.1. Adapted from figure found at Ritchie H, Roser M. Causes of Death. Our World in Data website. https://ourworldindata.org/causes-of-death. Published February 2018. Updated December 2019. Accessed January 11, 2021. Licensed under CC BY 4.0. Original figure based on data from Shen O, et al. Death: Reality vs. Reported. https://owenshen24.github.io/charting-death/.

health is often like: far from facts and far from foundational forces. It does not help that these forces tend to be complex, long-standing issues, while the topics we prefer to talk about tend to be new, simple, and easily absorbed into the partisan narratives that do so much to define the public conversation. A classic case in point for this was the pursuit of a vaccine for Covid-19. Now, finding a vaccine was by no means unimportant. But the race-against-time nature of the story, its focus on using the latest technologies to develop something new, its promise of the kind of breakthrough we have long accepted as a shorthand for scientific success—these are core points of interest in the stories we often hear about health. And they are the precise opposite of the stories we do not often hear but should—stories about long-standing, deeply rooted foundational forces that shape health.

A good way of looking at this is by way of an event that occurred near the beginning of Covid-19, on May 18, 2020. That day marked the fortieth anniversary of the eruption of Mount St. Helens. In reflecting on this event in the context of Covid-19, it is possible to see a parallel between the two emergencies. Both the eruption and the pandemic were sudden, acute crises that emerged from the slow shifting of foundational forces. In the case of Covid-19, these forces were what we have been discussing throughout this book—the structures that underlie our world and that can support health or open the door to disease, depending on their alignment. In the case of the eruption of Mount St. Helens, these forces were the literal foundations of our earth, tectonic plates changing their position over time. In each of these cases, slow shifts over a long period culminated in destructive events that captured the world's attention. Yet this attention is notably absent from the causes of such events as they unfold over the course of many years. How often, for example, do we hear news stories about the creep of tectonic plates in North America? It is not as though they no longer pose a threat. An eruption of the supervolcano beneath Yellowstone National Park, for example, could be a disaster of world-altering magnitude. Why, then, are there not nightly news stories about the potential causes of such a catastrophe? Because these causes are hard to see. Because the threat they pose seems too remote. Because there are other stories to distract us.

All this could be said of the foundational causes of a pandemic. Health can well be understood through the metaphor of plate tectonics. Every so often, we are hit with an eruption, like a pandemic, but until the moment they make themselves unignorable, we are content to keep looking away from the foundational forces that produce these events. Perhaps a reason the protests for racial justice surprised many is that they were an effort to engage with these forces, whereas in the past we have been all too willing to ignore them. This engagement was a truly radical step—not just because of the deep and multifaceted changes called for, but also because the protests were addressing foundational challenges with the urgency these problems deserve. In doing so, the protests were acknowledging that the time it takes for poor health outcomes to develop among marginalized populations is just as ripe for intervention as when these outcomes emerge into sudden, acute view. Those who could not equate the crisis of racism with the crisis of Covid-19 were not seeing the roots of poor health. Acute health challenges, although they seem sudden, are the result of the foundations of our world slowly shifting over the course of years, generations even. The difference is that while we can do little to address the structural forces that create earthquakes, we can engage with the foundations of health, centrally through the work of politics.

Politics may well be the most important foundational influence on health. Politics fundamentally shapes the distribution of the resources necessary for health. These resources include money, legal protections, the expectation of a level playing field in society, and the focus of public opinion, with its power to either alter or entrench the status quo. Politics decides whether our economy is fair or an unregulated Wild West. It decides how we address climate change. It can ensure equality before the law or skew our society toward injustice. Our engagement with foundational forces is shaped by social movements, corporate decisions, and the actions of groups and individuals, but it is arguably most fundamentally shaped by politics. Our political attitudes decide not just how we address problems but also whether or not we even see certain issues as problems at all. These perspectives are shaped by the political conversation, then codified into policy through the legislative process.

The centrality of politics was particularly inescapable during Covid-19 due to the fact that the pandemic coincided with the US presidential election. That contest contrasted two very different visions for the country and for our approach to the foundational forces that shape health. But the presidential election was not the only intersection of politics and the pandemic, nor was it necessarily the most important one. For decades, politics resulted in our government neglecting the foundations of health and declining to take the necessary steps to prepare the United States for the kind of pandemic we have known, ever since the days of SARS, would likely come. Our partisan battles have focused overwhelmingly on the immediate concerns of a given news cycle instead of on the long-term challenges we face. This shortsightedness has characterized thinking in both parties, and has had many decades to take root. Reversing course will take a reimagining of how politics addresses issues fundamental to health, which we will discuss at greater length later.

Covid-19 was a moment where the shifting of foundational forces created a crisis. We responded by engaging with these forces to mitigate, as best we could, worst-case scenarios. The ambition of federal-level economic relief, and the speed with which it was passed, showed government can pursue this engagement nimbly and with bipartisan initiative. The subsequent failure of the US government to continue acting boldly, until we had a change of federal leadership, highlights how often we fall short of acting on the forces that shape our health to the degree that we should. The protests for racial justice showed that we are capable of addressing the threat posed by the misalignment of these forces even when that threat is not apparent to everyone, even when some deny it exists. The protesters' engagement with the issue of racial justice soon resulted in a change in the political conversation, shaping the policies lawmakers were willing to consider and the trajectory of the presidential race. Preparing for the contagion next time will require even more of this engagement, as we widen our vision of what it takes to sustain health.

To do this, we need to look beyond medicine. During Covid-19, engaging with the foundational drivers of health was a matter of urgent necessity. This is no less true now. Even without a pandemic, we are faced with public health threats that are shaped by foundational forces. From the political and economic roots of the obesity epidemic and the social stigma that informs the opioid crisis to the many structural drivers of climate change, the social, economic, political, and demographic foundations of health are central to the challenges we must address, nationally and globally, in the years to come. Engaging with these forces helped inform our response to Covid-19; they can help us address these other challenges as well.

Just as a virus can have long-term effects on the body, the pandemic reshaped our societal foundations, with lasting implications for our economy, our culture, our attitudes toward core issues such as race, our politics, and more. In showing us what really matters for health and nudging us toward the steps we need to take to support a healthier world, the disaster of Covid-19 may yet yield some good. Whether the experience of the pandemic leads to significant long-term benefits will depend on whether we retain the hard lessons of that moment and apply them to foundational forces.

In her book *The Shock Doctrine: The Rise of Disaster Capitalism*, Naomi Klein advanced an idea with implications for the Covid-19 moment. She argued that large-scale traumatic events such as wars and natural disasters can, by radically upsetting the status quo, create space for self-interested actors to institute policies that benefit the powerful by exploiting populations affected by disaster. It is true that history provides no shortage of examples of this occurring. But the reverse is also true. Large-scale disasters, by exposing and upending the foundations on which societies rest, also create space for imagining radically new, radically better futures. Now that the pandemic has shown the areas where our foundations are cracked or misaligned, we are under no obligation to reassemble them the way they were before Covid-19. We should pursue new possibilities, built on foundations that can withstand any contingency. The Covid-19 moment showed how disasters can reshape our foundations; it also showed how a disaster is not the only force that can drive such change. Populations working together through social movements and the political process, motivated by the desire for health, can wield a positive influence that can turn even the legacy of a contagion into the makings of a healthier world.

5

Where We Live, Work, and Play

For most of us, the experience of Covid-19 will be forever linked to the details of a specific place. For those who were fortunate enough to be able to telecommute to work and leave the house only for short necessary trips to places such as the grocery store, this place was the home. The geography of the pandemic was the bedroom, the kitchen, the bathroom, the kids' play area, the living room, the hallway, and, in warmer months, the yard. Thinking back, we recall the moments of worry at our desks in whatever part of the house became our makeshift workstation, as we read online about the latest surge in cases. We remember the ritual wiping of the groceries in the kitchen after each trip to the store, as we did our best to ensure that our food was free of the virus. We think back on walks around the neighborhood, how we really *saw* those streets, as if for the first time, now that circumstances had forced us to limit our view to scenery we used to brush past on the way to wherever we considered more important. These details took on fresh meaning as we underwent a radically new challenge in the most familiar of spaces.

It is an irony of the pandemic that such a global event would have the effect of narrowing our scope of awareness to the people and places in our immediate vicinity. The more worrying the news from abroad, the more alarming the national scene, the more we looked to neighbors and local institutions for support. If the technological trends of recent decades have made the world feel closer than ever, the internet giving us a real-time feel for events anywhere on the planet, the pandemic returned us to a more local mode of existence—families living within small communities in a relatively limited geographic space. The physical layout of this space has always been important, but Covid-19 underlined this importance, making it central to our daily preoccupations. We needed our homes to be pleasant spaces because for months they were the only space we had. It was suddenly quite necessary for us to live in walkable communities, because going for walks was core to our ability to exercise in quarantine. Then there was the importance of social networks—real ones, not the dubious connections of social media.

My own experience of the pandemic was very much shaped by these connections. As dean of a school of public health, I was part of a group of people who were engaging with the pandemic at the local, national, and global levels as experts in the field of health, while also working to navigate the pandemic within the context of our campus. To ensure students could maximize their educational experience while respecting the requirements of safety, we reimagined the layout of our campus to align with physical distancing norms. We instituted limits on how many people could be in a room at a time; we put cameras in classrooms in service of a hybrid teaching model in which students could choose whether to come to campus or work remotely. These steps created a space that felt familiar yet different, which could well serve as a description of the whole world during the pandemic. At that time, we became even more conscious of community, of our good fortune to be working among supportive colleagues whose daily presence made those difficult months more manageable.

During the pandemic, I also, like so many, gained a new perspective on the place where I live. Throughout the lockdown, my family and I were subject to the same occasional doldrums as everyone else, but mostly we were imbued with a sense of gratitude for all we had. Seeing our home and neighborhood through the lens of the lockdown brought into focus the many ways place can function as a positive influence for health. We had ample space and food, means of telecommuting to work, a safe neighborhood near parks and places to walk, and a supportive network of friends and family. In thinking about these advantages, it became impossible not to consider those who do not have them, who live in places that undermine rather than support health. I thought of how sustaining it had been to be able to go for regular walks during the lockdown, and how it might have been different had we lived in a dangerous neighborhood. Or how much more challenging the lockdown would have been if my family of four had been confined to a small apartment rather than a spacious house.

Or how our social networks were key to our ability to navigate the pandemic, without which those long months would have been far more difficult.

At the same time, I thought of how the foundational forces discussed in Chapter 4 shaped my family's access to these advantages, of how much our experience of the pandemic was mediated by the conditions in which we live. My family was able to have an easier time of the pandemic because of the specific social, economic, political, and geographic contexts in which we found ourselves during Covid-19. If our neighborhood had been noisy or polluted, if our home had been run-down or too small, if our local political leadership had been lacking, such factors could have made the experience of Covid-19 significantly more challenging. On the other hand, when neighborhoods benefit from robust investment, when local leadership is competent and responsive, when homes are safe and comfortable, we are in a better position to weather crises than those living in places less conducive to health.

This chapter, then, is about place. Place is one of the key factors that determine whether or not we can live a healthy life, because of the simple fact that place is a ubiquitous exposure. It is what we encounter each day, shaping our lives and health. Covid-19 motivated us to think deeply about such exposures. Many of us likely still carry lists in our head from the days of the pandemic cataloging the places we regularly went and the level of risk we ascribed to those locations. This way of thinking was necessary for navigating the pandemic; it is also necessary for building a healthier world. We should always be thinking about how the physical spaces we navigate shape exposures that can either make us sick or keep us healthy. During the pandemic, this thinking helped us to avoid unnecessary risk. In a post-Covid-19 world, it can help us to conceptualize new spaces that actively generate health. This includes, principally, our homes and workplaces, the transportation infrastructure we use to get to and from these places, the towns and cities in which these journeys unfold, and the broader context of our global environment. This chapter will focus on how we can apply the new perspective on place afforded by Covid-19 to optimizing our world for better health. We will start with an overview of the link between place and health before focusing on the physical spaces where we live and work, our communities and transportation networks, and the condition of our global home. We will look at what Covid-19 taught us about the relationship of these places to health and how we might apply this knowledge to making the world a place where health can flourish and contagion cannot take hold.

When it comes to the influences that shape our health, there really is no place like home. Housing is fundamental to our ability to live healthy lives—indeed, it is fundamental to our ability to live at all. In his famous hierarchy of needs, the psychologist Abraham Maslow categorized, in order of importance, what he believed to be the factors necessary for human flourishing (Figure 5.1). Near the top of the hierarchy are higher-order goals such as self-actualization and feeling a sense of prestige and accomplishment. At the bottom—the level of basic needs—are the physiological necessities of food, water, and warmth. Our homes are where these core needs should be met. If they are not, if we lack warmth and security, then we will always be vulnerable to poor quality of life and the sickness that comes with it.

The first step to ensuring that homes meet basic needs is ensuring that people have homes to begin with. This means addressing the

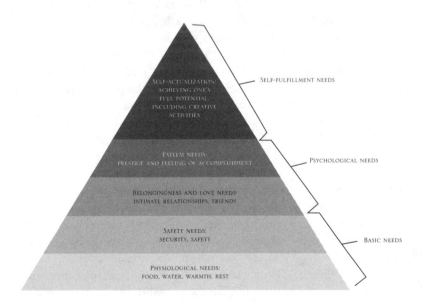

Figure 5.1. Adapted from figure found at McLeod S. Maslow's Hierarchy of Needs. Simply Psychology website. https://www.simplypsychology.org/maslow.html. Accessed January 7, 2021. Licensed under CC BY-NC-ND 3.0.

challenge of homelessness, a challenge that was worsened by Covid-19. At the school where I work, our community saw this firsthand. The Boston University School of Public Health is located in a part of the city with a high homeless population. During the pandemic, we heard many stories of how Covid-19 intersected with homelessness. One member of our community told of encountering a man who had managed to remain drug-free for months before he lost his restaurant job during Covid-19. Unable to afford his rent, he became homeless and started using drugs again.

Or there is the story of Kayvon, who spent months of the pandemic homeless because he could not afford first and last month's rent on an apartment. In an op-ed, he wrote about how his stimulus check was enough to keep him secure for about two weeks before he was back on the streets.

Such stories were not unique during the pandemic. Each speaks to the importance of addressing homelessness as a means of building a healthier world. But providing homes is not in itself enough to fully support health; it is merely a first step. Housing must then be of sufficient quality to create a context where health can thrive. There are many ways that substandard housing can undermine health. Residential units with poor ventilation can lead to the development of asthma. The presence of lead in a home can negatively affect mental and physical development in children. Dampness and mold can trigger allergic reactions and respiratory problems. Ventilation that can help mitigate these challenges was an important consideration at the time of the pandemic, as air quality in homes, schools, and workplaces became a priority issue. Ensuring proper ventilation was core to navigating the pandemic, but it is also core to our health at all times. If the physical spaces we inhabit each day are causing us to breathe unsafe air, what chance do we have of being healthy? Yet this is the reality faced by those who live in substandard spaces.

This challenge is worsened by the effects of crowding in housing units, which can aid the spread of infectious disease. In Chapter 1 we touched on the overcrowded, poorly ventilated urban tenements where diseases such as tuberculosis were able to gain a foothold at the start of the twentieth century. Homelessness, poor housing, and housing instability (roughly defined as spending over 50 percent of household income on housing) are all closely linked to the wider challenge of poverty. The key reason many people live in substandard housing, or do not live in homes at all, is because they lack the money to pay for a decent place to stay. This is why in discussing place and health, we must also discuss economic investment in communities. We cannot simply build quality housing while neglecting the neighborhood around it. Place means the full range of factors associated with where we live—our homes, yes, but also communities, local economies, and the link between these local conditions and the national investment that can improve them.

In the United States, place is also inextricably linked with race. This is perhaps reflected most explicitly in the legacy of redlining. The practice of redlining emerged in the 1930s, when the Home Owners' Loan Corporation—a New Deal–era program designed to help borrowers avoid foreclosure—made it semiofficial policy to segregate communities by drawing red lines on maps of cities to keep Blacks in one section and whites in another through discriminatory lending practices. This started a trend of disinvestment in many Black neighborhoods, creating conditions of poverty, lower educational performance, more exposure to pollution and extreme heat, and less access to parks and green spaces. With homeownership a key means of building intergenerational wealth in the United States, being consigned to such neighborhoods has helped undermine socioeconomic mobility in Black communities. All this has created a context where health cannot flourish as fully in many Black communities as it can elsewhere in the United States.

By delimiting where people of color can live, and ensuring that those places are often characterized by disadvantage, the legacy of redlining has helped keep race a central determinant of health in the United States. When we look at the many ways Black populations are less healthy than white populations, we are not just seeing health outcomes, we are seeing policy outcomes. We are seeing the downstream effects of policies such as redlining, which historically have created disadvantage manifesting as increased poor health for Black Americans. This poor health has long been a signal pointing to injustice, visible to anyone who cared to look, but during Covid-19 the signal was perhaps clearer than it has ever been.

In Boston, the city where I work, for example, the neighborhood of Roxbury was once given a red designation. In the years since, as the neighborhood has become home primarily to communities of color, the legacy of redlining has informed a pattern of disadvantage and poor health there, creating the conditions for acute challenge when the pandemic struck. During Covid-19, Roxbury was at significantly higher risk of Covid-19 than other parts of the city. It is sadly ironic that when Covid-19 cases would spike in a given area, those places were said to be "in the red zone." Given the history of segregation that has characterized communities of color, it could be said that these communities have been "in the red zone" for generations—ever since they were first assigned that color on the maps that excluded them from health.

The closer we look at who lives where, the more clearly we can see how housing is influenced by societal divides between those who enjoy the benefits of economic resources and social capital and the communities we have allowed to remain marginalized, cut off from the resources necessary for health. This is obvious when it comes, for example, to the line between the rich and the less well-off. Even individuals who are not disposed to think much about the lives of the poor cannot fail to see the stark difference between lower-income neighborhoods and the more privileged parts of a city or town. In this, the link between social marginalization, economic disenfranchisement, and housing inequality is all too clear. This is particularly true with regard to the historical roots of residential segregation and how they have concentrated the burden of this inequality within communities of color.

Covid-19 also showed where the link between place and social marginalization is perhaps less obvious, though not less significant for health, particularly health in a time of pandemic. One of the signature features of Covid-19 was the significantly higher threat it posed to a population we do not think about nearly as much as we should—older adults. A Kaiser Family Foundation analysis found that adults age sixty-five and older accounted for 80 percent of Covid-19 deaths in the United States. This age group already accounts for a sizable percentage of the US population and is fast increasing, driven by the aging baby boom generation. In 2018, there were approximately 52 million people in this age category in the United States; this number is projected to rise to 95 million by 2060.

These demographic shifts call for a radical reimagining of how our society treats older adults, including how it conceptualizes their living arrangements. Our current approach is often to let older adults become detached from the communities of which they have long been a part, consigning them to lives of physical isolation. Some cultures embrace the old, building family units around multiple generations living together in the same place, the young caring for their aging relatives and, in turn, receiving the benefits of wisdom and companionship. In the United States, however, we have accepted a model where older adults often live solitary lives, or else are sent to nursing homes where quality of care can vary widely. The concentration of older adults in nursing homes is an example of how societal values can shape the physical spaces in which we live. We do not yet value a model where older adults remain fully integrated into the community; our physical spaces reflect this by housing aging populations in facilities rather than homes. This was deeply significant during Covid-19, as nursing homes came to represent a front line of risk for those living and working at these places. As of March 31, 2021, at least 179,000 residents and workers in nursing homes and long-term care facilities had died from Covid-19, accounting for 33 percent of all Covid-19 deaths in the United States. The virus infected more than 1,345,000 people at about 31,000 such facilities, accounting for 4 percent of total US cases. As of December 4, 2020, at least half of Covid-19 deaths in thirteen states were linked to nursing homes (Figure 5.2).

This stark divide in Covid-19 mortality suggests a society that marginalizes its aging population, a marginalization reflected by place. We created the conditions for a concentration of older adults in facilities where the virus was able to gain traction, placing their health at elevated risk. Because of this risk, the measures necessary to protect aging populations meant isolating them even further, sealing off nursing homes from family and friends, whose visits are so important to supporting health, particularly at life's later stages.

How can we address housing with an eye toward improving health for everyone, young and old alike? The first step is properly investing in housing. We need large-scale federal investment not only to create affordable housing but also to create affordable housing of the highest possible quality. This means housing that is spacious, well-ventilated, and able to function as a home rather than as simply shelter. These homes should be embedded within neighborhoods that are likewise the beneficiaries of robust federal investment and policies that keep housing far from pollution and other hazards and close to walkable paths, green spaces, and opportunities for healthy recreation.

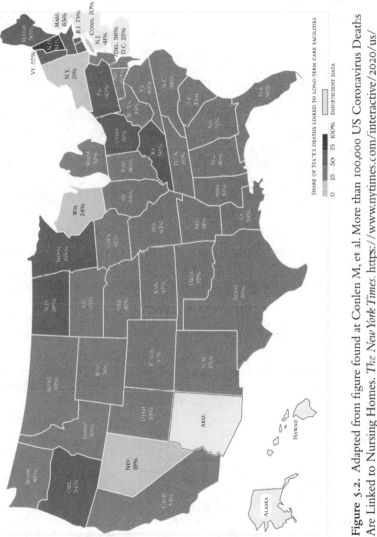

IN 13 STATES, AT LEAST HALF OF DEATHS ARE LINKED TO NURSING HOMES.

DATA AS OF DECEMBER 4, 2020

SHARE OF STATE'S DEATHS LINKED TO LONG-TERM CARE FACILITIES

0   25   50   75   100%   INSUFFICIENT DATA

Figure 5.2. Adapted from figure found at Conlen M, et al. More than 100,000 US Coronavirus Deaths Are Linked to Nursing Homes. *The New York Times.* https://www.nytimes.com/interactive/2020/us/coronavirus-nursing-homes.html. Updated December 4 2020. Accessed January 8, 2021.

I am aware that in calling for greater federal investment in housing I am taking a side in a contentious debate. Many would argue housing is best handled at the community level, with local governments working with private developers to ensure that a percentage of new housing is affordable while letting the market drive the construction and design of these spaces. This engagement is indeed important; partnerships between the public and private sectors can yield much good toward creating a healthier world. However, the scale of the project called for if we are to truly meet housing needs in this country can only be comprehensively supported through a large-scale federal initiative. This is a country that has used the full mobilization of its resources to win world wars and help rebuild the countries they affected. It has put human beings on the moon. It maintains a defense budget of staggering proportions. Our limits are not on our resources but on our imagination. The task of adequately housing everyone in the United States is equal in scale and urgency to prior initiatives. But while we have found ourselves capable of imagining moonshots and wars, we have been less able to imagine a true commitment to national housing. This failure of imagination has excluded millions from the basic conditions of warmth and security necessary for health. We are a country that is endlessly concerned with the higher-order needs in Maslow's hierarchy, such as prestige and self-actualization. Yet we have neglected the foundational needs that enable their pursuit. Allowing everyone to pursue a life characterized by true well-being means first ensuring that the basics are taken care of, basics such as housing. This cannot be accomplished through a patchwork of public-private partnerships. Rather, we should view housing the same way we view education—as a condition so key to a healthy citizenry that it justifies the federal spending necessary to make it accessible to everyone living in this country.

This is not to say that the design and construction of housing should be left entirely to the state. A national push for universal housing would take federal funding, yes, but the creation of new living spaces could be a truly multisector initiative. Building spaces that maximize livability and health would draw on expertise from architects, artists, and public health professionals and engage with community-level input to ensure that new units meet local needs. These needs would, of course, vary. What would work in, say, Tulsa would not necessarily work in Chicago. Yet there are some principles—good ventilation, access to green spaces, handicap accessibility, and so on—that work anywhere and are worth embracing widely.

Housing is core to health for the simple reason that our homes are where we spend much of our time. We are constantly exposed to the conditions of home; if those conditions are conducive to health, we are likelier to stay healthy, and if they are not, we are likelier to get sick. But there is another place where we spend significant amounts of time, in some cases even more time than we spend at home: the workplace. Our workplaces are central to our health, both as the places where we earn our living and as where we encounter the exposures that shape our health. During Covid-19, these exposures were most often defined as the interpersonal encounters that could lead, potentially, to exposure to the virus. Early in the pandemic, a divide emerged between workers who were able to minimize this risk through telecommuting and those who were unable to do so. The latter were often in low-wage positions with little flexibility—fast-food workers, for example. This meant that the divide between those risking the most and those risking the least, in terms of potential Covid-19 exposure, often aligned with existing economic divides. For workers lacking the option to telecommute, the issue of workplace exposures was now at top of mind. While before Covid-19 it was possible to progress through a career without ever thinking about how the physical character of the workplace might be shaping health, during the pandemic every possible exposure was cause for concern. Workers needed to think about the number of people they encountered on a given day, where they encountered them, and how the risk inherent in those encounters might be mitigated. They were forced to consider the physical layout of their workplaces: Was there enough space for social distancing? Was there proper ventilation? Did the employer take special precautions, and were there laws in place to require such measures? It became clear that the physical layout of where we work can mean the difference between sickness and health. It was also clear how many of the factors that determine whether or not workplaces are healthy are out of the hands of individual employees. Even employees who were able to telecommute still had to think about this; it was this very consciousness of risk that shaped their choice to stay home.

Working conditions have shaped health throughout history, as have the social movements that have sought to improve them. In his 1906 book *The Jungle*, Upton Sinclair wrote about the dangerous and unsanitary conditions in the meat industry. The book helped change the conversation around workplace safety and led to many of the reforms of the Progressive Era. While workplaces are now significantly safer than they were before such reforms, places of employment remain areas of potential danger. In 2018, there were 5,250 fatal work injuries recorded in the United States; these included fatal transportation injuries, incidents involving contacts with objects and equipment, and fatal slips, falls, and trips. In addition to the unique hazards associated with certain lines of work, workplaces are shaped by the same range of conditions that affect residential spaces, such as pollution exposure, poor ventilation, and neighborhood quality.

Just as reforms improved working conditions in the Progressive Era, social movements and legislation can improve conditions in the post-Covid-19 era. This includes creating safer working spaces and maximizing the health-promoting effects of time spent in these spaces by raising the minimum wage. Workers should not have to place themselves at risk to earn a living, nor should that living ever be less than enough to support a fully healthy life. But ensuring that workspaces are not actively hazardous to health is just the beginning. Workspaces should be places that *generate* health, places that are every bit as supportive of health as homes. To mitigate risk of infection, the pandemic necessitated a radical rethink of the physical layout of workplaces. Many workplaces rose to the challenge, altering their physical space in the name of health. We should not lose this willingness to make changes to our workplaces toward the goal of better health. Whether this means altering the physical space to make it safer, providing on-site childcare to help working parents strike a better balance between their jobs and their family life, fostering greater diversity and inclusion in the workplace, or working toward a spirit of mutually supportive community among employees through training exercises and staff outings, there are many steps we can take to ensure that the hours we spend at work unfold in the healthiest possible context.

Then there are the places that take us from place to place—the transportation infrastructure, which carries us to and from work, errands, vacations, visits to family and friends, and all the other destinations that lend richness and variety to life. Americans spend hours each day in cars and on planes, trains, and buses. Before Covid-19, our thinking about a given mode of transportation was generally limited to the question "Will this get me where I want to go on time?" If we thought about transportation's intersection with health and safety, it tended to be about limiting the incidence of catastrophic accidents. As long as our modes of transportation were not egregiously unsound, we were content to not think much about how they were shaping our health.

Covid-19 changed this. Our reliance on transportation networks and their influence on our health became an issue of core importance during the pandemic. Carefully weighing the risks of taking the bus or train to work, calling a cab or an Uber to visit a friend, or flying to another state to be with family for the holidays, many decided these journeys were simply not worth the potential danger. Others, however, lacked the choice to opt out of travel, placing the link between transportation and health at top of mind for the millions trying to get where they needed to go during the pandemic, despite potential exposure to the virus.

It is important to remember that the vehicles carrying us are themselves destinations, spaces we inhabit, just as subject to the broader conditions that shape health as any settled place. Our engagement with these conditions can help create a healthier status quo for all modes of travel. We have already achieved notable success in doing so in the area of road safety. The twentieth century saw a 90 percent decrease in road deaths between 1925 and 1997. The reason? Seatbelts, anti-drunk-driving laws, education campaigns to promote road safety, better-designed vehicles—in short, changes at the corporate, political, and cultural levels that reshaped the context of driving to make it safer. We saw inklings of this comprehensive approach to healthier transportation during Covid-19, as companies adopted new practices to make our journeys safer. While this was happening, many states adopted restrictions on travel, imposing quarantine and Covid-19 testing requirements on travelers from out of state, deepening our collective investment in healthier transportation. While, fortunately, we have moved beyond a need for such travel restrictions, we should not move beyond a commitment to shaping healthy transportation networks.

Transportation networks also shape health within communities, particularly urban communities. Situating a bus depot in an urban neighborhood can, for example, improve quality of life there by giving residents easier access to other parts of the city. But it can also generate unhealthy pollution, as can a major highway that cuts through a residential area. A train station can help residents commute, but the noise it makes can also disrupt their sleep and add to stress. Urban living can provide easy access to trains and roads, but in some places it can be inhospitable to walking or biking. Integrating transportation into urban spaces in ways that support health is part of the broader challenge of shaping healthier cities.

With the large, and growing, number of people living in cities, the way we design and run urban spaces has become central to the future of health. During the pandemic, the link between cities and health was inescapable. With their high concentration of people, cities were often epicenters of the virus. This created even deeper challenges for cities, as the public health crisis led to economic uncertainty.

For example, in New York City, which was at one point the pandemic's epicenter in the United States, Covid-19 disrupted momentum behind the opening of Hudson Yards, a $25 billion mixed-use private development project—the largest such project in American history. The twenty-eight-acre Manhattan development—with shops, housing, office space, restaurants, and the highest sky deck in the Western Hemisphere—was designed as the peak in urban living and luxury. Kael Goodman, president and CEO of the real estate data analysis firm Marketproof, was quoted in the *New York Times* as saying, "Hudson Yards is in some ways disconnected from the city—it's a city within a city, and it's operating at a global scale." For all the project's ambition, it could not escape the uncertainty caused by Covid-19, which left its commercial and residential space empty enough to cast doubt on its ability to be an immediate economic boon to New York City.

The woes of Hudson Yards reflect a shortcoming in how we think about cities, one with implications for health. Creating "a city within a city" tailored to high-end demand reflects an approach to urban development that relies heavily on building rarified spaces that cater to the wealthy but are less accessible to everyone else. These spaces are successful as revenue-generating ventures for the city, and they certainly facilitate healthy living for those able to afford such workplaces and homes. However, pouring money and design talent into making one or two dozen acres into the city of the future for the benefit of the very few can distract from creating the city of the future for the benefit of the many. One of the reasons Covid-19 was able to bring life to a halt in so many cities is that urban spaces are not yet designed with health in mind. They are patchwork configurations, with some neighborhoods enjoying lavish investment, some coping with neglect, and all subject to shifting political and economic imperatives, which, when they do align to benefit health, tend to do so only incidentally. When a pandemic strikes, it is the worst of all possible worlds. The disease is able to take root in more socioeconomically vulnerable neighborhoods, then spread until it has paralyzed the entire city, threatening even the most well-off members of the community and stymieing economic production across the board.

In the post-Covid-19 world, we have an opportunity to take a radically different course. Urbanization is a signature trend of the twenty-first century: urban spaces are evolving fast, new cities are rising, and these changing currents can be channeled in a healthier direction. With cities in flux, now is the time to create urban spaces that maximize health based on a vision of the public good. Doing so allows us to apply the understandings of housing, workplaces, and transportation discussed in this chapter to the creation of new skylines that signal health. Cities are perhaps the ultimate ubiquitous exposure. To live in a city is to be fully immersed in the factors that give it its physical and social character. These factors are uniquely able to be influenced by the kind of thoughtful, data-driven engagement that shapes a healthier world. Cities are home to large numbers of people living in a relatively small space. Nearly everything about this space save the weather is human-made, making cities uniquely malleable, with the potential for being shaped into whatever we would like them to be. If we were to design cities with health as their main organizing principle, we could turn them into some of the healthiest places on earth. Redlining showed we can engineer cities for the worst; we can also engineer them for the best—for health—if we so choose. To exponentially improve health in the twenty-first century, we need to be willing to leverage the lessons of these times into building urban spaces that are fully walkable, home to parks and green spaces, characterized by widely accessible quality housing, free of pollution, and easily navigable via cutting-edge transportation networks.

Creating such cities will not be possible unless we recognize that our shared health depends on our shared space. It is not enough to develop high-end spaces within cities and think the revenue they generate can substitute for building cities that support the health of everyone. A key lesson of Covid-19 is that no place is immune to poor health when we have not invested in creating a healthy world for everyone.

This calls to mind "The Masque of the Red Death," a short story by Edgar Allan Poe. The tale takes place in a time of plague and tells of the efforts of a group of nobles to escape the contagion by sealing themselves in an opulent abbey, believing themselves secure in their safe space. This security proves to be an illusion, however, as the plague somehow finds its way into their hideout, where it decimates their gathering until no one is left. Grim as this story is, it is also instructive. It illustrates that the only way to create spaces that are free of disease is to create a world where everyone, not just a select few, can be healthy. Had the nobles in Poe's tale invested their energies and fortunes in building a world that was truly healthy, their fate might have been different. We need to invest in making the world a place where everyone can enjoy the best possible health.

Covid-19 showed us that, for all the segregation in our society, for all the difference between high- and low-income neighborhoods, for all the variety of spaces we navigate, there is really only one *place* to truly speak of—the world we share. The story of place and health is ultimately the story of how we can support the long-term sustainability of our planet and maximize health. Just as it is not enough to have nice homes if they are situated in dangerous neighborhoods, it is not enough to make our communities more conducive to health if we neglect the broader environmental challenges that shape the health of our fragile, indispensable world. This means, centrally, mitigating the effects of climate change by designing healthier, more sustainable cities (even as we tackle the root causes of the climate crisis).

In June 2020, the *New Yorker* ran an article by Kyle Chayka titled "How the Coronavirus Will Reshape Architecture." The piece explored how other contagions, such as tuberculosis, may have influenced how we design buildings, and how Covid-19 might have a similar influence on our physical spaces. Disease has shaped place throughout history, from the cholera outbreaks that informed the development of modern street grids (with straighter roads to accommodate new sewage systems) to zoning laws designed to minimize the crowding that can give rise to disease in cities. Whether and how Covid-19 will exert a similar influence remains an open question. There has already been speculation that the rise of telecommuting might render large office buildings obsolete, as working from home becomes more of a settled norm. It is also possible to imagine a widening of city streets, or shared spaces in general, to promote physical distancing. These innovations are important and represent one component of how design can be a force for promoting health. However, we should not limit our engagement with place after Covid-19 to some design tweaks and a greater acceptance of telecommuting. We need to enlarge our imagination about what place can be, how it can maximize health and minimize the inequalities that currently characterize so much of where we live, work, and play.

6

Politics, Power, and Money

Of all the people to contract Covid-19, the most famous was likely US president Donald Trump. Trump was reported to have tested positive for the coronavirus in early October 2020. This diagnosis came soon after a White House event announcing Trump's nomination of Judge Amy Coney Barrett to the Supreme Court. Following the event, several attendees in addition to the president tested positive for the virus. It was an event at which, notably, many of the guests did not wear protective masks or practice physical distancing. In this, they were acting in accordance with the tone set by Trump, who rarely wore a mask during the pandemic and expressed skepticism about the effectiveness of face coverings. This skepticism helped to make mask-wearing into a partisan flashpoint as the pandemic unfolded. This was of a piece with the president's tendency to, at times, downplay the severity of the virus and the threat it posed to health. A recording of the president from March 2020 captured him saying to the reporter Bob Woodward, "I wanted to always play it down. I still like playing it down. . . . Because I don't want to create a panic."

The president's approach to the virus did not so much lessen public concern as polarize it. Covid-19 struck about three years into the Trump administration. A divisive figure since practically the moment he emerged on the national political scene, Trump was, by the start of 2020, someone in whom many Americans believed either completely or not at all. This had the effect of making the issues with which he engaged into matters of left-right political conflict, and the pandemic was no exception. Trump's attitude toward addressing Covid-19 transformed what could have, should have, been seen as basic public health measures into fraught political issues. Masks became a symbol of this polarization. Wearing a mask was seen by many as a mark of opposition to the president, while taking a less cautious approach to Covid-19 was seen as signifying support for Trump.

While mask-wearing eventually became less polarized as the pandemic wore on, there was a moment when Democrats were much likelier to report wearing a face mask or face covering than Republicans. An ABC News poll, reported in April 2020, asked respondents if they had worn such coverings in the past week when leaving home. Sixty-nine percent of Democrats said yes, while just 47 percent of Republicans said yes. Democrats were also likelier than Republicans to report worrying about the virus and making changes to their lives in response to the disease. This included changing travel plans, working from home, and supporting government policies that quarantined people who traveled to affected areas, canceled large gatherings and long-distance travel, and closed schools and universities (Figure 6.1).

Even the president's own hospitalization with Covid-19 was not enough to reverse the politicization of the virus. This was made abundantly clear upon Trump's return to the White House after his treatment at Walter Reed National Military Medical Center. He left Walter Reed wearing a mask, but when he returned to the Executive Mansion, he promptly walked up the stairs to the South Portico entrance and removed his face covering, posing for the cameras for about two minutes before walking inside the building, all while likely still being infectious.

The political divide during Covid-19, with some Americans painstakingly adhering to mask-wearing and physical distancing while others behaved as if times were more or less normal, was a striking example of how politics shapes attitudes toward health. It was by no means the first example of such a divide. Politics has long influenced how we engage with the conditions that shape health. Perhaps the example most analogous to the polarization of attitudes about Covid-19 is partisan engagement with the issue of climate change. When it comes to climate change, the science is clear: the earth is warming and humans are the cause. As we have already discussed, extreme weather events in the climate change era pose a threat to health, as do many other aspects of climate change. This raises the importance of large-scale action to mitigate what climate change has already done and to prevent the worst of what it might still do. In the United States, however, differing political opinions about the causes and scope of the climate crisis have rendered the subject intractably

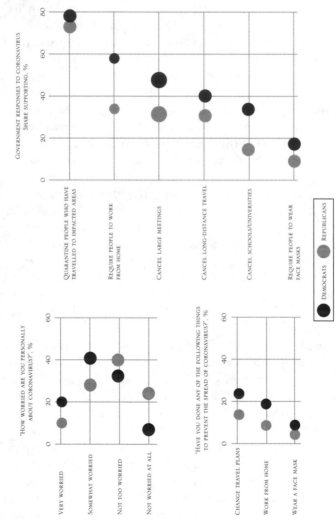

Figure 6.1. Adapted from figure found at In America, Even Pandemics Are Political. *The Economist.* March 11, 2020. https://www.economist.com/graphic-detail/2020/03/11/in-america-even-pandemics-are-political. Updated March 12, 2020. Accessed January 6, 2021. Figure data source: YouGov/*The Economist.*

partisan. The Democratic Party has largely accepted the science concerning climate change and the need to address this challenge, while the Republican Party has largely rejected these points. This has transformed what should fundamentally be an issue of scientific agreement (or disagreement) into a political one and has hindered our country's ability to engage with the issue, placing health at risk.

The polarization of opinion about Covid-19 reflects a broader truth about the pandemic: our experience of the crisis was deeply shaped by politics. This was due in part to the unique historical moment in which the pandemic unfolded—the run-up to the 2020 presidential election. During the latter half of any election year, politics are difficult to avoid, but the tenor of the Trump era contributed significantly to this politicization in 2020. With such a polarizing figure in the White House, and with the rise of social movements in reaction to the Trump agenda, the years leading up to Covid-19 had left much of America crouched in partisan corners.

But the election and daily politics of the Trump era were not the only way politics colored our experience of the pandemic. The fact that politics is so often conveyed to us through the real-time filter of the media can obscure the fact that politics' influence runs far deeper than the effects of a given news cycle. Politics shapes and is shaped by underlying social, economic, cultural, and geographic forces. It unfolds across time and is best viewed from a historical perspective. Seen through the lens of history, it becomes apparent that key political outcomes are the result of decades, even generations, of changes to a society, which culminate in watershed moments such as the election of a president, how a society handles a pandemic, or the state of a nation's health at a given point in time. Over time, politics—the actions of political leaders, the rise and fall of various ideologies, and the emergence of social movements—creates the context for our daily lives.

Politics shapes this context, centrally, by shaping the allocation of resources in society. Who will have housing? What groups will the rules of our economy favor? Who reaps the full benefits of citizenship and whose share is only partial? Fundamentally, all these questions then become a single question: who gets to be healthy? Housing, money, jobs, equality before the law, social inclusion—such factors are all necessary conditions for health.

Politics is the nexus at which these factors intersect. Just as the forces that shape health converge to a unique, highly concentrated degree in cities, the capacity to make decisions that influence these conditions converge to a unique degree in politics. Other areas where high-level decision-making matters for health, such as the corporate world, still do not have as much power to influence health as the world of politics. Returning to a previous example, the tobacco industry has significant power to shape the health of populations. Its choice to aggressively tar-get global markets has consequences for health in every country where tobacco companies operate. But the tobacco industry does not enjoy an entirely free hand to pursue its profits as it sees fit. Governments can choose to regulate the industry, or exclude certain businesses from the market altogether, through legislation. Political leaders can use rhet-oric to shape public attitudes toward tobacco use. Indeed, if political leaders can motivate their supporters in the midst of a pandemic to reject protective masks, then they wield a persuasive capacity even the most sophisticated corporate marketers might envy. As powerful as an industry such as tobacco may be, then, it is still subject to the control and influence of politics.

This, of course, invites the rebuttal that corporate interests can just as easily assert control over the political process through the use of money. Contributing to political campaigns to buy influence over pol-iticians has indeed long been a means of shaping political outcomes. But the very necessity of such tactics speaks to the ultimate centrality of politics as the arena where the key decisions are made affecting our lives and health.

This includes decisions about the economic conditions in which we live. As we have discussed, there are some tasks too big to be under-taken outside of government. These include the regulation of the sys-tems of finance that influence the levels of fairness or inequality in our society. Economic inequality is a key driver of poor health; this was particularly true during the pandemic, when the poor were much like-lier to suffer than the rich. Politics can reduce this inequality or worsen it by creating or withholding economic regulation. Indeed, it could be said this is the true heart of money in politics. It is significant that money can buy political access, but it is arguably even more significant that politics can help to mitigate economic inequality or deepen the already wide gap between those with more money and those with less.

It is for all these reasons that preventing the contagion next time has to involve working at the intersection of politics, power, and money. The pandemic revealed just how influential these forces are in creating a society that either supports health or undermines it. This chapter will explore these forces, looking at how politics and power shape health outcomes, with special emphasis on how these forces intersect with economic inequality and the disproportionate burden of sickness experienced by low-income populations.

From almost the moment it emerged, the spread of Covid-19 was shaped by politics. This began with politics within China, as the government worked to address the disease. It then became a global political issue, as governments and international bodies such as the WHO calibrated their response to the threat. Finally, it became an issue for US politics when the disease arrived on our shores. At that moment, American political leadership faced a test of its ability to respond to sudden crisis. Addressing a pandemic is a political task on par with any of the large-scale challenges a government can face. Rising to such a difficult occasion requires detailed plans for what to do in such a scenario, robust public health infrastructure, and leadership that takes decisive, data-informed action, listening to experts, and communicating clearly and consistently with the public.

Tragically, Covid-19 found the United States lacking in all these areas. The pandemic was a disaster, in the manner of a hurricane or earthquake. No matter what, it was going to cause some measure of poor health. But also like a natural disaster, the pandemic was predictable, and there were steps we could have taken at the political level to prepare for it. We cannot know when hurricanes will come, but we know they will come, and so we build levees, we fund the Federal Emergency Management Agency (FEMA), we create detailed playbooks for what to do when storms strike, and, when they arrive, we do all we can to support the experts as they work to mitigate the disaster. Likewise, we could not know when a pandemic would occur, but we knew one likely would at some point; it was therefore incumbent on our political leadership to do everything possible to ensure that it could not be said that a single death was due to the government not doing something it should have done, either in its preparation for a pandemic or in addressing the crisis as it occurred.

Unfortunately, the Trump administration largely failed this test. The problem was bigger than Trump's personal willingness to downplay the virus. Far worse was his willingness to ignore and at times vilify public health experts, as well as the sheer inconsistency of his administration's approach to the crisis. Public health depends on good communication between health authorities and the populations they serve. The public needs to feel it can trust the people giving them advice about that most crucial of matters—their health. When that trust is lacking, public health professionals cannot be fully effective in their work. It does not matter if the advice is sound and data-driven; if people do not believe it, then it will be of diminished use. The key to establishing trust is communicating with clarity and consistency. If public health messaging changes, it should be because the data changes, not because political expediency seems to demand it. Throughout this communication process, it is important that health authorities are supported by the words and example of those in positions of political power.

This process did not proceed smoothly during Covid-19. During the crisis, public health authorities worked at the local, state, and federal levels to provide accurate, up-to-date information to the US population. These efforts were frequently undermined by the Trump administration—specifically, by the erratic, undisciplined, and capricious words and actions of the president. In addition to his refusal to consistently model best practices for ensuring safety—instead spurning masks, continuing to hold large rallies, and permitting a culture of laxity around the virus within the White House itself—the president was often at odds with health experts and the broader, self-evident reality of the situation. A notable example of this was during the October 22, 2020, presidential debate, when President Trump claimed that the country was "rounding the turn" on the virus. At the time, the country was, in fact, experiencing an uptick in cases. The gulf between the tone set by the president and the reality of the pandemic created unnecessary problems for the health authorities trying to promote an accurate perspective of the crisis and take effective steps to address it.

This speaks to the key role of communication and rhetoric in shaping politics' influence on health. It is a role that is at times overlooked. When we think of political power and the means by which it affects health, we are liable to think first about the policies that shape our priorities and investment. Policy is certainly important, but the ability to shape public opinion is arguably just as important a political tool as working through the legislative process to achieve a desired outcome. Abraham Lincoln said, "Public sentiment is everything. With public sentiment, nothing can fail; without it, nothing can succeed. Consequently he who molds public sentiment goes deeper than he who enacts statutes or pronounces decisions." Public opinion is what can give an idea the necessary momentum to become policy. Political leaders are in a position to mold public opinion, nudging the public mind toward new ways of thinking.

The precise term for this is "shifting the Overton window." The Overton window is named after political thinker Joseph Overton (Figure 6.2). It refers to the range of topics considered acceptable for the mainstream political discourse. Subjects that fall within the Overton window can be discussed in the public conversation without the stigma of seeming extreme. Subjects outside the window are seen as varying degrees of radical, and at the far end of the spectrum they are unthinkable. When a subject has entered the Overton window, this mainstream acceptance brings it one step closer to becoming settled policy

An example of this is the issue of same-sex marriage. Just thirty years ago, same-sex marriage was regarded as outside the realm of

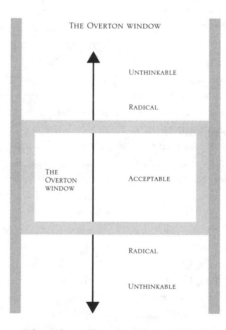

Figure 6.2. Adapted from figure found at Pigott J. The Overton Window: Some Thoughts . . . *Medium.* April 17, 2018. https://medium .com/@julianpigott/is-it-good-to-have-an-overton-window-11a6acb0884c. Accessed January 7, 2021.

possibility—not just among its conservative opponents but among many in the LGBT community. As recently as fifteen years ago, national candidates in the Democratic Party, a party that now includes LGBT rights as a central part of its platform, would not voice public support for marriage equality. But in the last decade and a half the conversation changed, the Overton window shifted, and acceptance of same-sex marriage went from being mainstream among the American public to being mainstream among politicians to being mainstream among a Supreme Court majority that made marriage equality the law of the land.

In the case of marriage equality, the Overton window was largely shifted by changes in public opinion about same-sex marriage, with political leaders following the evolving attitudes of constituents. This was the case, for example, with Barack Obama, who earlier in his political career expressed ambivalence about, and occasional opposition to, same-sex marriage before ultimately voicing support for it as president. Obama's public evolution on the issue roughly paralleled the country's evolution over a twenty-year period toward greater acceptance of the LGBT community and greater willingness among Americans to insist political leaders support the rights of this population.

However, political leaders do not always follow the public in shifting the Overton window. They also possess the unique power to move it themselves. President Trump proved particularly adept at changing the conversation, pushing it to new extremes. This was his effect during Covid-19, when his statements and actions undercutting public health helped shift norms around how Americans engaged with the pandemic. By helping to mainstream a cavalier attitude toward Covid-19, the administration shifted the Overton window toward greater acceptance of behaviors that create poorer health.

In the fall of 2020, Columbia University Earth Institute's National Center for Disaster Preparedness published a report titled "130,000–210,000 Avoidable COVID-19 Deaths—and Counting—in the US." As the title suggests, the report found that by that point in the pandemic, between 130,000 and 210,000 deaths could have been avoided in the United States with better political leadership. These findings should, of course, be viewed cautiously. During Covid-19, such studies were always subject to a degree of uncertainty, and they are best seen in the context of the broader body of knowledge about the disease. However, it is also the case that most experts have suggested that we

could have avoided deaths by addressing Covid-19 earlier and better. The Columbia report arrived at its conclusion by comparing the
country's political response to Covid-19 and its death toll from the
pandemic to that of comparable high-income countries. In looking
at these countries—Japan, South Korea, Canada, Germany, Australia,
and France—the report found that if we had embraced the measures
they adopted, our pandemic outcome might have been very different.
These measures include an earlier lockdown, increased testing capacity, the federal government providing clearer guidance on social distancing, and a national mask-wearing mandate. The slow and at times
incoherent response of the Trump administration, with its failure to
take key steps to address the pandemic, was found to be a significant
reason the United States saw such disproportionately high mortality.

Around the time of the Columbia report, the editors of the
New England Journal of Medicine published a piece titled "Dying in
a Leadership Vacuum." The editorial strongly criticized the Trump
administration's response to the pandemic, citing its failures as a key
reason for the country's high Covid-19 mortality, and going so far as
to say, "Anyone else who recklessly squandered lives and money in this
way would be suffering legal consequences." This condemnation was
all the more striking for appearing in *NEJM*—a journal that is more
than two hundred years old and which as a rule does not make political statements of this kind. The mission of the journal is to contribute
to a body of knowledge that generates health. That it should have
been moved to make such a pointed critique of the administration's
handling of the pandemic speaks to the close link between political
leadership and health, and how catastrophic it can be when such leadership is lacking.

It is important to mention here that politics does not invariably
mean Trump. In discussing the political response to Covid-19, it is
impossible not to focus on the actions of the Trump administration.
However, as we will discuss, the political forces that shape health
during a pandemic transcend a given administration. Nevertheless, the
actions of specific leaders at a specific time and place do matter. To
return to the ship metaphor with which I started the book, the leader
is the captain. She or he is at the helm, and much depends on the
assuredness with which the vessel is steered. Yet the condition of the
ship itself (our public health infrastructure) is also of primary importance, as is its direction (our overall approach to health). This chapter is

centrally concerned with the actions of the captain, but we must never lose sight of the other elements at play that shape our voyage.

Covid-19 was a time when foundational forces intersected with the decision-making of specific political actors to shape health, and, indeed, to shape the course of world history. But it was not the only time this happened. In 1918, an influenza pandemic was raging. In about fifteen months, it killed between 50 and 100 million people worldwide. In the US alone, the disease killed approximately 675,000 people. Yet Woodrow Wilson, who was president at the time, made little effort to address or even acknowledge the crisis. World War I was under way, and Wilson appeared concerned that discussing the pandemic would hurt morale and possibly undermine the war effort.

But just because the Wilson administration was inclined to ignore the virus does not mean the virus ignored the administration. Paralleling what was to occur almost exactly a century later in the Trump White House, Wilson's efforts to downplay the virus took place even as the pandemic touched the president's inner circle. Wilson's daughter and secretary were infected with the flu, as were multiple members of the Secret Service—even the White House sheep were said to be infected. In another historical parallel, the president himself would catch the disease—at a moment of deep historical significance.

In 1919, Wilson arrived in Paris for peace talks to establish the trajectory of Europe in the wake of World War I. It was around this time that he became sick with influenza. While Wilson's staff played down the president's condition, the truth was that the president was violently ill with the disease. He was so sick that people close to him observed he was never the same after his experience with the flu. Not only did the disease appear to influence Wilson's personality, but it may have influenced the all-important peace negotiations. Wilson had earlier argued that the victorious Allies should be lenient toward the defeated Germans. Wilson was hoping to lay the groundwork for his brainchild, the League of Nations. Easier terms for the Germans could have helped inform the spirit of international cooperation necessary for starting the League off on the right foot, to ensure it would be able to keep the peace in the years to come. However, other voices at the talks argued for taking a harder line with Germany. After his bout with the flu, Wilson reversed course on the matter and did not stand in the way of a more punitive approach to Germany, one so harsh that it arguably set the stage for the nationalism and resentment that would inform the rise of Adolf Hitler and the outbreak of World War II.

Would Wilson have continued advocating leniency for Germany had he not been physically debilitated by influenza? It is impossible to know. What is clear is that the actions of individual leaders are a key mechanism by which politics affects the conditions that shape health. Had Wilson acted differently during the peace talks, history could well have taken a different turn, possibly away from the recurrence of global war. That Wilson was in a position to influence this trajectory was a function of the political process which elevated him to power. When we engage with this process, we play an active role in shaping who is in the room when decisions that affect our health are made. Will these political actors share our values? Will they have the level of competence necessary to lead effectively in times of crisis? The answers to these questions are vital to health, and they are decided by politics.

The intersection of the Wilson administration and the influenza pandemic was an example of how pandemics shape history, and how failure at the political level to fully address contagions when they occur is, sad to say, nothing new. Wilson's hesitance to acknowledge a pandemic has been shared by subsequent presidents, from the Reagan administration's slowness to name and address HIV to the Trump administration's downplaying of Covid-19.

Yet it would be unfair to lay blame for ignoring disease solely at the feet of political leaders. The truth is that we have collectively downplayed the conditions that shape health, and we have done so for decades. In refusing to consistently treat Covid-19 with the seriousness it deserved, the Trump administration was sharing in a shortcoming for which we all bear some responsibility. When it comes to ignoring the conditions that made us vulnerable to the pandemic, we have, as a society, been just as negligent as some of our leaders.

Perhaps the central example of this is our failure to adequately address race in the United States. We have neglected to reckon fully with the effects of racial injustice in this country—in particular, its effect on health. The pandemic revealed this failure for all to see. The racial injustice the pandemic and protests exposed encompasses not just the experience of interpersonal racism, or even the experience of police brutality. It goes deeper, revealing fundamental inequity. This inequity reflects the need for political solutions to the problem of racism. Just as political leaders in the 1960s recognized that promoting racial justice was inextricably linked to ensuring voting rights for Black Americans, addressing this injustice in the present will take a politics that addresses foundational issues such as housing segregation, the racial wealth gap, and other reflections of systemic injustice.

Among the factors that shape health, the area of race is particularly sensitive to political dynamics, where the words and actions of political leaders can have outsized influence on the public debate. For progress to be made, political leaders must listen and speak with empathy, guided by a willingness to understand how systemic injustice has placed health out of reach for communities of color. Instead of just muddling through to get to the next news cycle, leaders must engage with moments of acute challenge around race, having the political courage to name the societal failures these moments reflect.

A key example of this was in the immediate aftermath of the assassination of Martin Luther King Jr. in 1968. As word of the murder spread, some American cities experienced rioting as anger about the assassination spilled into the streets. At this fraught moment, Senator Robert Kennedy, who had recently declared his candidacy for the presidency, spoke to a low-income, predominantly Black neighborhood in Indianapolis. Many in the audience had not yet heard the news about King. Kennedy told them about the murder, and tape of the speech conveys their shocked reaction. Kennedy—who rarely, if ever, publicly referenced the death of his brother President John F. Kennedy—then spoke from his personal experience about the temptation to feel hatred over such an act. Continuing, he addressed the root causes of the country's fraught racial history:

> What we need in the United States is not division; what we need in the United States is not hatred; what we need in the United States is not violence and lawlessness, but is love and wisdom, and compassion toward one another, feeling of justice towards those who still suffer within our country, whether they be white or whether they be black.

There were riots in more than a hundred cities the night Kennedy gave that speech, but there was no rioting in Indianapolis. Historians have credited Kennedy's words with helping to keep the peace there at that difficult time. Central to the speech's power was its call for justice and compassion as fundamental tools for addressing the causes of violence—the violence that took King's life and the violence that occurred in response to this crime. It spoke to the universal human values from which good policy emerges, policy that truly makes a positive difference for health.

At its best, politics can address the foundational forces that under-lie our health or leave us open to disease. It can bring attention and clarity to these issues, elevating challenges the public conversation has neglected and rallying support for finding solutions to the key prob-lems we face. It can also recognize when social movements are already doing this work organically and marshal support for these forces. Ideally, politics and social movements operate in a complementary manner, with leaders in positions of power channeling activist momentum into good policies while helping to cultivate an even broader base of public support for these ends.

There are few better uses for this momentum than addressing one of the key drivers of poor health in the United States: the gap between those who have the most money and those who have significantly less. Money buys the basic standard of living necessary for health. It provides a cushion in times of crisis, helping individuals, families, and communities weather the storms of contagion, economic downturn, or, in the case of the Covid-19 moment, both. Americans lacking these resources felt the weight of the pandemic much more, and for much longer, than more economically secure segments of the population. What is more, the pandemic did much to increase the number of peo-ple experiencing financial strain. Between February and April 2020, 10 percent of Americans between the ages of twenty-five and fifty-four lost their jobs (Figure 6.3).

While the economy recovered toward the summer of 2020, this recovery was not shared equally. For high-wage workers making over $60,000 per year, employment rates rose to a level nearly on par with rates before the crisis. However, employment remained much lower for low-wage workers, those making less than $27,000 per year (Figure 6.4).

The recovery was also segregated by race, with Black Americans recovering a little over a third of lost employment, while white Americans recovered over half in the early months of the pandemic (Figure 6.5).

All this had the effect of making the recession caused by Covid-19 "the most unequal in modern US history," in the words of a *Washington Post* headline. This is particularly clear when we compare

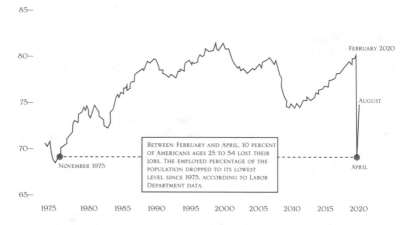

PERCENT OF PEOPLE 25–54 WHO ARE EMPLOYED

BETWEEN FEBRUARY AND APRIL, 10 PERCENT OF AMERICANS AGES 25 TO 54 LOST THEIR JOBS. THE EMPLOYED PERCENTAGE OF THE POPULATION DROPPED TO ITS LOWEST LEVEL SINCE 1975, ACCORDING TO LABOR DEPARTMENT DATA.

Figure 6.3. Adapted from figure found at Long H, Van Dam A, Fowers A, Shapiro L. The Covid-19 Recession Is the Most Unequal in Modern US History. *The Washington Post.* September 30, 2020. https://www .washingtonpost.com/graphics/2020/business/coronavirus-recession- equality/. Accessed January 7, 2021.

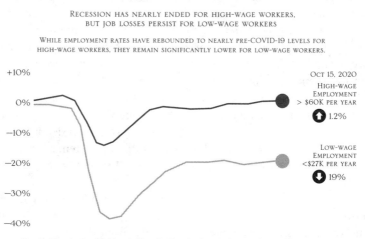

RECESSION HAS NEARLY ENDED FOR HIGH-WAGE WORKERS, BUT JOB LOSSES PERSIST FOR LOW-WAGE WORKERS

WHILE EMPLOYMENT RATES HAVE REBOUNDED TO NEARLY PRE-COVID-19 LEVELS FOR HIGH-WAGE WORKERS, THEY REMAIN SIGNIFICANTLY LOWER FOR LOW-WAGE WORKERS.

Figure 6.4. Adapted from figure found at Opportunity Insights Economic Tracker. Track the Recovery website. https://www.tracktherecovery.org/. Accessed January 10, 2021.

PERCENT OF PEOPLE WHO ARE EMPLOYED

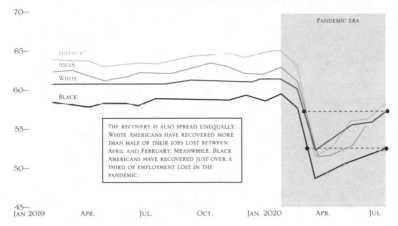

Figure 6.5. Adapted from figure found at Long H, Van Dam A, Fowers A, Shapiro L. The Covid-19 Recession Is the Most Unequal in Modern US History. *The Washington Post.* September 30, 2020. https://www .washingtonpost.com/graphics/2020/business/coronavirus-recession-equality/. Accessed January 7, 2021.

the Covid-19 recession to previous economic downturns. While in past recessions everyone was in roughly the same economic boat, during Covid-19 the experience was dramatically different for high- and lower-income groups. Those with more money experienced relatively little disruption, quickly bouncing back from unemployment. Those with less money, however, lost jobs that largely did not come back, creating the conditions for permanent economic hardship (Figure 6.6).

Covid-19 may have been the driving force behind the recession, but it did not create this inequality, nor the racial injustice with which this inequality intersects. That long predated the pandemic. In 2018, a Black woman named Pamela Rush traveled from Alabama to Washington, DC, where as part of the Poor People's Campaign she testified before US lawmakers on poverty in her county and the predatory lending practices that helped prevent anyone in the region from climbing out of it. In her testimony she said, "They charged me over $114,000 on a mobile home that's falling apart. . . . I got raw sewage. I don't have no money, I'm poor." Two years later, she died from Covid-19.

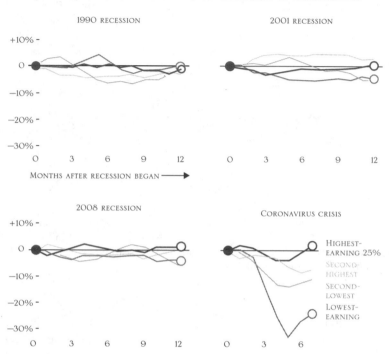

Figure 6.6. Adapted from figure found at Long H, Van Dam A, Fowers A, Shapiro L. The Covid-19 Recession Is the Most Unequal in Modern US History. *The Washington Post*. September 30, 2020. https://www .washingtonpost.com/graphics/2020/business/coronavirus-recession-equality/. Accessed January 7, 2021.

Her death is inseparable from the conditions in which she lived and in which millions of her fellow Americans live. The gap between those with the most money and those with less has increasingly become a gap between the healthy and the sick. Exclusion from economic stability is exclusion from health—full stop. It is difficult, if not impossible, to lack access to the resources that support health and still manage to live a healthy life. Figure 6.7 reflects this. It draws on research led by economist Raj Chetty that found that between 2001 and 2014,

LIFE EXPECTANCY BY INCOME QUARTILE BY YEAR

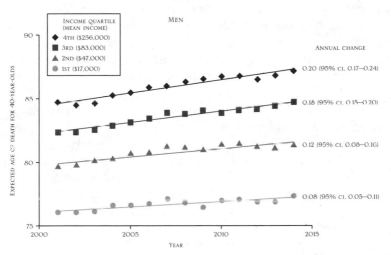

CHANGES IN RACE- AND ETHINICITY-ADJUSTED LIFE EXPECTANCY BY INCOME GROUP, 2001 TO 2014. | JAMA

Figure 6.7. Adapted from figure found at Belluz J. What the Dip in US Life Expectancy Is Really About: Inequality. *Vox.* https://www.vox.com/science-and-health/2018/1/9/16860994/life-expectancy-us-income-inequality. Updated November 30, 2018. Accessed January 7, 2021.
Original figure data from Chetty R., et al. The Association Between Income and Life Expectancy in the United States, 2001–2014. *JAMA: The Journal of the American Medical Association.* 2016; 315(16): 1750–1766.

Americans at the top of the economic ladder gained about five years of life expectancy, while Americans at the bottom gained none.

This gap is closely intertwined with race. In 2020, I was part of a research team that looked at racial/ethnic differences in depression rates among US adults. We found that lack of socioeconomic assets explained some of the differences in depression risk between Black and white adults. If we do not consider socioeconomic assets at all, we see higher depression rates reported among Black adults. But when we take differences in these assets into consideration, we find that both Blacks and Hispanics appear to have better mental health than non-Hispanic whites. This difference is not entirely a matter of money—it also reflects social factors such as marital status—but it speaks strongly to how finances are central to the experience of poor health outcomes.

Addressing the economic inequality and systemic racism that informs health divides is the work of politics. Pamela Rush knew this when she traveled to Washington, DC. She went there because she understood the problems of her community to be so deeply entrenched that only the power of the federal government could fully address them. As long as our politics does not engage with these challenges to the necessary extent, we will remain vulnerable to the next pandemic. When Rush spoke before lawmakers in 2018, no one could have known that a pandemic would strike just two years later. But it would have been easy to predict that, in the face of such a disaster, communities sharing the disadvantages Rush experienced would have been likely to suffer most. To end this vulnerability for good, we need to follow Rush's lead and engage at the political level with the intersection of race and economic disadvantage. This will take a politics that supports federal spending and is not afraid to embrace redistributive economics in service of investing in communities.

In particular, this investment must address where historic racial injustice meets economic inequality, and this involves addressing the racial wealth gap. The average Black family controls approximately $10 in assets for every $100 controlled by the average white family. This reflects generations of economic and social disadvantage, and no intervention can be fully effective without addressing this historical context. For this reason, we need a politics bold enough to pursue policies that engage with this history. At the heart of these policies should be a national plan for reparations paid to the descendants of slaves, both to materially support the advancement of Black communities and to acknowledge, as a nation, the systemic roots of the disadvantage these communities have faced.

Reparations are, admittedly, controversial, as is the level of public spending necessary to address the socioeconomic roots of poor health. But much has shifted in recent years, including public opinion on key issues such as race. It is the task of politics to help shift opinion still further, changing minds as prelude to changing policy. Figure 6.8 is a visualization of the common trajectory of social movements. It reflects how movements can spring up after an initial triggering event, enjoy a "honeymoon phase" of maximal public engagement, then start to taper off after substantive change is perhaps not immediately forthcoming. There is then a process of learning and reflection, followed, ideally, by regrowth of the movement. Covid-19 was a classic triggering event,

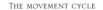

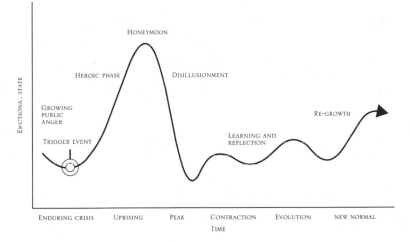

THE MOVEMENT CYCLE

Figure 6.8. Adapted from figure found at Saavedra C. Five Ways Funders Can Support Social Movements. *Stanford Social Innovation Review.* July 9, 2018, https://ssir.org/articles/entry/five_ways_funders_can_support_social_movements. Accessed January 7, 2021.

bringing to light societal shortcomings that left us vulnerable to a pandemic. These problems require political solutions. During the pandemic, there was movement toward these solutions, from addressing the economic roots of poor health to a reckoning with racial injustice. We are now far enough removed from the pandemic that we risk losing some of this momentum. This is understandable. We are all tired after the trauma of Covid-19; it makes sense that we would want to simply drop the issues raised by the contagion, embrace a return to the pre-Covid-19 status quo, and abandon the project of systemic change. This is understandable, but it is not acceptable. The next outbreak could be worse than Covid-19, and when it comes, we must be ready. Being ready means applying the lessons of the recent past to creating a healthier future.

Keeping these lessons at top of mind is the task of politics. Strong political leadership can help social movements maintain momentum, channeling public attitudes into policies that support health. This task may seem dauting, but political engagement is, by nature, an often laborious process, its most significant outcomes the culmination of much work. As the sociologist Max Weber put it, "Politics is a strong and slow boring of hard boards." It takes ambition combined with patient commitment to creating the structural changes that shape a healthier world. As difficult as this work can sometimes be, it is not possible to build such a world without political engagement. There is simply no substitute for politics.

SECTION 3

The Values That Should Inform These Conditions

7

Compassion

During Covid-19, our engagement with the pandemic was at times complicated by the challenge of stigma. For example, early in the crisis, awareness of the pandemic's Chinese origin occasionally led to the scapegoating of people of Asian descent. In a piece for *Scientific American*, Connecticut doctor Jennifer Tsai wrote about this:

> In the Emergency Department, a patient's father halts me with a fanned palm a foot from my chest—prevents me from examining his child even though I've introduced myself as the doctor—and inquires if I've "been home recently." My ability to take care of a gasping boy is questioned on account of my Taiwanese ethnicity. A week later, a triage nurse asks a new patient why he has come to the hospital. He responds, simply, that he had recently been "coughed on by [an] Asian."

Stigma affects our health in a range of ways, in this case potentially preventing a child from receiving needed care. In Chapter 2, we discussed how stigma has complicated our approach to addiction, obesity, and mental health in the United States. More broadly perhaps, stigma has interfered with our ability to think clearly about the origins of disease and what to do about them. At core, we are still deeply invested in the idea of individual culpability for disease. When we see someone who is sick, we are tempted to assume that person did something to deserve it. Perhaps we do not always frame this thinking in such accusatory terms; however, we remain wedded to the idea that health is a product of the individual's lifestyle, and this is a short step from attributing even infections from a novel virus during a pandemic to the individual, implying it was their fault they were infected. On a day-to-day basis, when we encounter someone suffering from, say, obesity or addiction, there is a temptation to ascribe these challenges to personal shortcomings, such as lack of self-control, rather than to the structural forces that truly shape health.

This thinking has a long history, which is revealed in the study of past epidemics. When the Black Death reached Europe in the fourteenth century, the continent faced a catastrophic threat about which it knew very little. In the absence of modern science, populations had to cope with the physical, social, economic, and spiritual effects of the disease with scant understanding of what it was, where it came from, or how it might be stopped. Many theories filled the gap created by this lack of knowledge, including the notion that those suffering from the plague deserved it—that it was God's punishment for sin. This belief informed the practices of a religious group called the Flagellants. Members of the group believed the ravages of the plague were God's judgment for human error. As a form of penance, the Flagellants would roam from village to village, whipping themselves bloody. Their movement had existed prior to the arrival of the plague, but the experience of contagion helped grow their ranks, their activity supported by the idea that if populations could sufficiently atone for whatever they did to deserve the plague, the contagion might finally relent.

As archaic as the practice of the Flagellants may sound to us now, their vision of personal culpability for poor health is not far from our own willingness to stigmatize individuals for getting sick. And while the acts of the Flagellants may have been brutal, were they any more brutal than when we refrain from taking policy steps that could make people less sick because we regard poor health as somehow deserved? I would argue that this policy violence, while less lurid than the brutality of the Flagellants, is every bit as medieval in its vision of the moral acceptability of letting the "culpable" pay dearly for disease. When we deny vulnerable populations quality health insurance, when we refuse to expand Medicaid, when we play political games with the social safety net, when we suggest that government programs helping the disadvantaged somehow incentivize poor life choices among these groups, we are applying a tone of judgment that would not be out of place in a medieval morality play.

This feeling of judgment is something to which we are all susceptible, and it cuts across social and political divisions. For example, it is not uncommon to hear it expressed in the mainstream conversation—a conversation amplified by the media—that a core challenge to creating a healthier world is conservative opposition to the social safety net. This opposition is often motivated by the notion that those who have lived healthier lives should not have to subsidize the care of those who have become sick as a consequence of their own poor decisions. It is also possible to sometimes see blame directed toward the socio-economically marginalized—the population most likely to need the safety net—for voting against leaders who support policies that generate health. Why, it is sometimes asked, does this demographic vote against its own interests? It is not difficult to detect, as subtext to this question, a hint of judgment toward these voters, and an implication of their culpability for any sickness their electoral choices bring to communities.

But the question we must really ask ourselves is what is truly worse for health in the long run—the voting habits of a given group, or the human tendency to judge and scapegoat others? It is likely true that the majority of voters simply wish to care for their families and live decent lives, and they support candidates they feel, rightly or wrongly, will help them do so. This impulse strikes me as being far more conducive to the long-term sustainability of a healthy society than the impulse to judge these people. Instead of judgment, we need compassion, a willingness to see the world from other points of view, and, when we feel it is indeed necessary to work toward a change in political attitudes, the resolve to do so from a place of respect rather than recrimination. Such compassion was often lacking in the Covid-19 discourse. Had it not been so lacking, had we applied compassion to all we did during the pandemic, our response to the crisis might have been very different.

The national response to Covid-19 was colored by partisan fault lines that often shaped our attitudes toward those who became sick. During the pandemic it was not uncommon to see news stories reporting Covid-19 infections among recent attendees of Trump-supporting events where mask-wearing was less than rigorously observed. When, for example, former presidential candidate Herman Cain was diagnosed with Covid-19 and later died from the virus, it was often reported that he had recently attended a Trump rally where he did not wear a mask. Now, lack of masks at such events and the resulting infections were well worth reporting on, both as newsworthy events and as cautionary tales for the rest of the population about what not to do during a pandemic. But an honest assessment of how we related to each other during the pandemic cannot fail to miss a slight quality of judgment toward the infected whenever it was clear they had not taken the right steps to protect themselves, a judgment that seemed all the sharper when it was made from the other side of the political divide.

It is perhaps simply human nature to think this way. Is this any different from when we hear that someone we know had a heart attack and we think, "Well, she was obese"? Or when we hear someone died of lung cancer, and think, "Well, she was a smoker"? Partisanship can amplify this sentiment, but it need not be informed by political animus or the hyperreligious fervor of the medieval Flagellants to take root. It simply reflects a truth about the human condition: we are all fragile, finite, and vulnerable to anything that can happen in a chaotic, dangerous world. The truth of our existence is that misfortune can and will befall us no matter what we do. To judge someone for their poor health is to respond to this vulnerability by implying that we, as individuals, have more control over our health than we actually do. It is to deny the larger forces that shape our lives and health. We cast judgment to avoid the truth that, outside of engaging with these forces, there is actually little any of us can do as individuals to ensure the expectation of health throughout our lives. Stigma then emerges from our evasion of this fundamental truth. We insist on others' culpability to avoid thinking about our own vulnerability.

This is not to say, of course, we should remain neutral about the choice to not wear a mask during a pandemic, only that it is possible to discourage such recklessness while also eschewing the feeling of judgment that is the antithesis of compassion. This reflects how the challenge of poor health presents a fork in the road. One path can lead us ever deeper into fear and a willingness to express that fear by projecting it onto others through stigma and blame. The other path can take us toward compassion and the better world compassion can create. We saw glimpses of this world even amid Covid-19. The experience of weathering a shared public health threat pushed us toward each other—in solidarity, in grief, in active engagement with each other's lives. This was informed by a new spirit of mutual understanding. We knew how our neighbor was feeling because it was how we were feeling. We all worried about ourselves and our loved ones. We all felt the frustration of the moment. We all wondered when the crisis would finally end. These shared feelings helped counter the stigma and judgment that occasionally emerged during the pandemic. Even as we were exposed to some of the uglier pathologies to which societies can give rise, we were shown a vision of how compassion represents a path out of crisis.

But compassion is more than a lifeline at difficult times. It can be a guide for building a better world, one that is free of contagion. Compassion helps us to see the structures that underlie poor health, and it motivates us to do something to improve them. This is because when we experience compassion fully, we find we cannot look away from the circumstances that characterize the lives of the people around us. This thinking inevitably leads to a reckoning with the forces that shape these circumstances. We recognize, through compassion, that if we truly care about others, if we truly wish to support their well-being, we cannot fail to address the context in which they live. Compassion necessitates a confrontation with the gap between the world as it is and the world as it could be. Had compassion been the animating force behind all we did during the pandemic, we might still have disagreed about the right steps to take, but we would have done so without the animus that so often characterized these conversations, and with our eyes fixed not on the depth of our disagreements but on the shared context that shapes our health.

The importance of compassion was reflected in an article that ran in *STAT News* early in the pandemic about the challenge of caring for the homeless population in San Francisco. Few interactions are more generative of compassion than engagement with the homeless. The article detailed the steps taken by the city and by individual caregivers to pursue this engagement during Covid-19. These included using local hotels to help the homeless isolate and letting some people with nowhere else to go stay in hospitals, even if their symptoms happened to be mild. These all represent acts of compassion in the face of challenge. They also reflect how compassion is inextricably tied to the basic public health measures necessary for protecting the whole population, not just the most vulnerable. The defining feature of infectious disease is that it spreads; compassion for the vulnerable in times of contagion, then, is also compassion for the population at large. A world in which the homeless can be healthy is a world in which everyone has a better chance of avoiding preventable disease. Without working toward such a world, our efforts to support the health of others will always be incomplete.

This was the case in San Francisco, where those looking to care for the homeless soon found there were limits to what they could do. None of the steps they took on behalf of the homeless, however effective, solved the main problem—homelessness itself, and the societal structures that help create and perpetuate it. This problem was well summarized by Margot Kushel, director of the Center for Vulnerable Populations at the University of California, San Francisco, who said, "Covid-19 is making clear what we have always known—that underlying structural conditions leave those most vulnerable at highest risk." This is where compassion ultimately points—to the structural forces that generate hardship in the first place.

In San Francisco, compassion for the homeless led first to a simple recognition of the challenges faced by this vulnerable population, then to an embrace of steps toward addressing these challenges, then to a recognition of the limitations of these steps within the framework of existing structures. The next step is a reckoning with the structures themselves. There is a logic to this progression, an equation that compassion forces us to acknowledge if we are to create lasting solutions to poor health in our society. To see poor health through the eyes of compassion is to see past individual behaviors and into the context that creates poor health. If compassion is able to bring us to this point, it is a small leap indeed to go from perceiving these challenges to actively engaging with them. In stirring the compassion of so many, the pandemic set our society on a path that can lead us to an understanding of what must be done to build a world that is truly healthier. The fundamental ask of this book is that we look beyond the confines of the crisis to see that putting out the fires of Covid-19 is not enough as long as the conditions that set them remain in place. Compassion helps us to see this broader reality and motivates us to change it.

In this way, compassion reveals the centrality of values to our approach to health. So far in this book, we have discussed what could perhaps be described as the more tangible aspects of building a healthier world. We have talked about the fundamental forces of history, politics, money, and place. Just as fundamental, however, are the values that inform our engagement with these forces. These values include compassion, the pursuit of social and economic justice, and the understanding that health is a public good. If the direction of our ship is our collective approach to health, our values could be called the stars by which we navigate. They help us to set our direction and steer through the climate of uncertainty and historical contingency that character-izes any effort to fundamentally change the world. In making the case for the importance of values, this book joins other voices that have long been calling for a focus on values as a guiding force for action. These voices include Donald Berwick, a former administrator of the Centers for Medicare and Medicaid Services, who in an article for *JAMA* titled "The Moral Determinants of Health" wrote, "Healers are called to heal. When the fabric of communities upon which health depends is torn, then healers are called to mend it." Such work takes more than scientific knowledge—it takes values that guide meaningful action within societies, with compassion at the forefront.

Like stars, values are all the more important when times are dark. It is precisely when we face moments of challenge that values such as compassion can provide direction to see us through difficulties. During the pandemic's early days, when we were faced with a sudden, unprecedented crisis, it was difficult to know what to do. Compassion helped move us forward, reminding us of our basic obligation to care for others. In coming together to aid the most vulnerable, we were able to see a way through those months of challenge. Even when it seemed like there was no end in sight, compassion provided a structure for our actions during the pandemic. We might not have always known what the next day would hold, but we knew that when it came, acting with compassion toward others would always be the best step to take, the surest way to get to a better, healthier future.

When institutions and governments are guided by a similar frame-work of values, they have on hand a reliable means of parsing potential courses of action and deciding on the ones that maximize well-being. Compassion can help them recognize the measures that most effec-tively engage with the conditions that shape health. A compassion-ate view of homelessness, for example, helps us to see the realities of economic uncertainty, housing insecurity, addiction, and social stigma that together are the reason so many live on the streets. Policies that support health, then, are policies that help to improve these conditions. Crucially, compassion shows how no single factor is responsible for poor health—it is the interplay of conditions in our society that creates challenges such as homelessness. So in addition to suggesting policies that can address poor health in populations, it also elevates the fact that policy response must take the form of multiple initiatives, with no single law or program a panacea.

This approach is by no means intuitive. We like to think there are simple solutions to our problems—a pill we can take, a behavior we can modify, a candidate we can vote for—that, once embraced, will close the book on our challenges. This is particularly true when it comes to disease, where our priorities have long favored the search for cures rather than the more difficult business of preventing disease by addressing the complex web of factors from which sickness emerges. In the policy space, preventing disease means addressing poor health on multiple levels. Homelessness, for example, should be addressed at the intersection of housing, addiction recovery support, and economic justice. This solution can be difficult to see, but compassion helps us to do so, providing an important example of how values help us make sense of complexity and help us envision a healthier world.

This section of the book, then, will address values, and their central role in preventing the contagion next time. We start with compassion because it is arguably the foundational value for building a healthier world. We all understand the need for compassion, we all feel compassion for others, and we all have had our eyes opened, at various times in life, to the societal challenges that compassion reveals, challenges that stand in the way of health. During Covid-19, compassion showed us just how many people in the United States are deeply vulnerable to poor health. As we have discussed, this vulnerability was often a product of underlying health conditions. This was clear early on, as data out of China showed the Covid-19 death rate to be higher for populations with underlying conditions such as chronic respiratory disease, cardiovascular disease, and diabetes (Figure 7.1).

The emergence of this information—that certain groups were at higher risk of Covid-19—helped inspire compassion among the broader public as we came together, collectively, to care for the vulnerable. Yet these data can also create the impression that, even during a pandemic, it is possible for socioeconomic advantage to allow certain segments of the population to avoid our common risk. When we believe this, we are then able to believe that poor health is only a challenge for "those people," for the marginalized and disadvantaged groups whose lives are already likelier to be characterized by stigma and poor health. It is important not to let this impression take hold. Compassion is rooted in an understanding of our shared humanity. It comes when we recognize that when anyone is unhealthy, we are all at risk of being unhealthy, so we need to create a context where no one

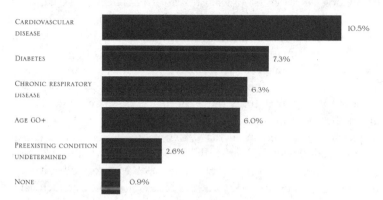

Figure 7.1. Adapted from figure found at Whyte LE, Zubak-Skees C. Underlying Health Disparities Could Mean Coronavirus Hits Some Communities Harder. NPR. April 1, 2020. https://www.npr.org/sections/health-shots/2020/04/01/824874977/underlying-health-disparities-could-mean-coronavirus-hits-some-communities-harde. Accessed January 6, 2021. Figure data source: Chinese CDC. Credit: Talbot R, Zubak-Skees C.

faces this risk. The experience of an infectious threat can be a powerful reminder that our health is linked. There are many health challenges in the United States that annually generate a level of mortality comparable to that of Covid-19, challenges such as obesity and addiction. However, we have not addressed these challenges with anywhere near the level of urgency we brought to bear in addressing Covid-19. A key reason is, arguably, that these challenges are not infectious, making it possible for the public at large to escape the visceral feeling of vulnerability to a disease that transmits through the air and can strike anybody. Instead, we see these challenges somehow as niche issues, the niche being the lives of people who lack advantages. This outlook allows us to evade the feeling of common humanity that gives rise to compassion.

Compassion, then, depends on the understanding of the true nature of health and of our shared vulnerability to disease. During Covid-19, this vulnerability was heightened by the media environment. Covid-19 was the first global pandemic of the social media age, an era that coined the phrase "going viral" to describe the sudden, rapid spread of information across communication platforms. This context amplified anxiety in the face of contagion, keeping concerns about the virus front and center and helping ensure that for many the fear of the disease was never far from mind.

While such constant anxiety is never desirable, and in the case of Covid-19 likely contributed to the significant increase in depression rates observed at that time, the experience of shared risk did help inform the spirit of compassion that emerged during Covid-19. Yet compassion grounded in media-driven anxiety is not a sustainable means of building a healthier world. The media climate during Covid-19 helped keep us informed and supported a level of collective concern that indeed motivated us to care for each other. But such care is most durable when it is rooted in a deep understanding of the forces that generate health, forces that should be every bit as central to our thinking about health as Covid-19 was at the height of the pandemic.

We have throughout this book explored how these forces created vulnerability for certain populations during Covid-19. These populations happened to be older adults and people with preexisting conditions. I say "happened to be" because there is much about the disease's evolution that was random. Figure 7.2 is based on a chart made early in the pandemic, comparing Covid-19 symptoms to those of cold and flu. A key challenge of the pandemic was disentangling the signs of Covid-19 from those of other sicknesses. Figure 7.2 clarifies why this was so difficult. Cold, flu, and Covid-19 shared many overlapping symptoms, including headache and cough. To make matters more confusing, as our experience with Covid-19 unfolded, it became clear the virus presented in sometimes dramatically different ways, with a range of odd symptoms and long-term complications. Whereas at one point it seemed to be primarily a respiratory challenge, it later appeared to affect, in some cases, the heart and brain.

The many and varied symptoms of Covid-19 reflect the randomness with which viruses evolve and affect populations. Likewise, the fact that Covid-19 was more dangerous for certain people was entirely a matter of chance. We should therefore be careful about making broad assumptions about our society's resilience in the face of pandemics based solely on who was able to escape this latest contagion. That socioeconomic advantage was able to somewhat insulate segments of the population from the worst of Covid-19 does not mean such

SYMPTOMS OF THE COLD VS. FLU VS. CORONAVIRUS, AS
SUMMARIZED BY NATIONAL INSTITUTE OF ALLERGY
AND INFECTIOUS DISEASES

	SYMPTOMS	COLD	FLU	COVID-19
	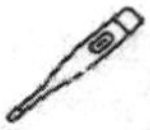 FEVER	RARE	HIGH (100–102 F)	COMMON
	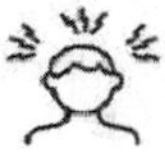 HEADACHE	RARE	INTENSE	CAN BE PRESENT
	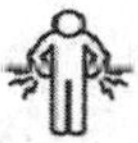 GENERAL ACHES, PAINS	SLIGHT	USUAL, OFTEN SEVERE	CAN BE PRESENT
	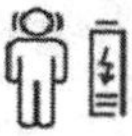 FATIGUE, WEAKNESS	MILD	INTENSE, CAN LAST UP TO 2–3 WEEKS	CAN BE PRESENT
	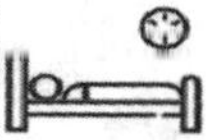 EXTREME EXHAUSTION	NEVER	USUAL (STARTS EARLY)	CAN BE PRESENT
	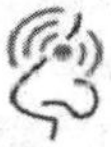 STUFFY NOSE	COMMON	SOMETIMES	HAS BEEN REPORTED
	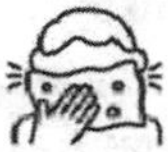 SNEEZING	USUAL	SOMETIMES	HAS BEEN REPORTED
	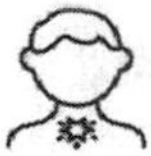 SORE THROAT	COMMON	COMMON	HAS BEEN REPORTED
	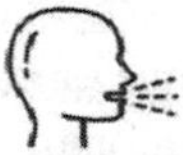 COUGH	MILD TO MODERATE	COMMON, CAN BECOME SEVERE	COMMON
	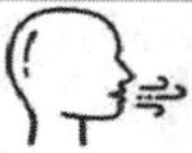 SHORTNESS OF BREATH	RARE	RARE	IN MORE SERIOUS INFECTIONS

Figure 7.2. Adapted from figure found at Symptoms Chart: Cold, Flu or COVID-19? *Cottage Grove Sentinel.* March 16, 2020. https://cgsentinel.com/article/symptoms-chart-cold-flu-or-covid-19. Accessed January 6, 2021. Figure data sources: National Institute of Allergy and Infectious Diseases. CDC. WHO.

advantage is invariably protective during pandemics, only that it was during this particular one. Even so, the disease still managed to spread to the most privileged among us, infecting even the president.

The next pandemic will likely be no less arbitrary in its symptoms and its victims. We cannot know in advance what it will do or whom it will most affect. It could exclusively kill children, people with blond hair, the obese. For all we know, you, the reader, could be the next unknown's ideal victim. For this reason, we should not forget our initial feelings about the pandemic, when we did not know whom it would harm or to what extent. In one sense, for all the damage caused by the pandemic, we escaped the worst of what might have occurred. In another, we are never beyond the reach of the worst-case scenario. As long as we accept a world where contagion can take hold, we remain at risk of a virus emerging that sweeps through the population, killing millions, hundreds of millions, or even more. Because we all live with this threat, we should have compassion for each other, recognizing we are in the same boat, as we work toward a world without this risk.

I say this not to frighten but to motivate. I want to motivate us, collectively, to look at health through the lens of compassion, because it is the right thing to do. Not just right in the moral sense, but right in terms of being the only practical way we can build a society that is no longer vulnerable to poor health. This starts with discarding the distinction between "your" health and "mine," and realizing that when we tolerate the conditions that create poor health, when we use stigma to avoid thinking about the true causes of why certain people get sick, we are building what is ultimately a trap for ourselves. We may manage to avoid the trap for a long time—so long, perhaps, that we start to forget it is there, or assume we are too advanced, too wise, too rich, too socioeconomically insulated to ever fall into it. Then comes an acute challenge—it could be a worldwide pandemic, or it could be the more commonplace realities of aging, sickness, misfortune, and the slide into death that all humans face—and suddenly we are exposed to the flimsiness of the illusion, and to the truth that the only way to create a world where these realities can be managed is to create one where everyone can access the resources necessary to do so.

Looking at health with compassion is in many ways a radical step. Not just in the way we typically define "radical"—that is, as calling for a fundamental restructuring of society for the benefit of the common good. It is radical in the deeper sense of addressing health not only at the level of economics, society, and politics but also at the level of simply being human in a chaotic, dangerous, but also infinitely improvable world. Covid-19 showed us it does not matter if one is rich or poor. We all have in common the human condition, and part of that condition is vulnerability to sickness. And when pandemics come, even if we do not fall into the category of the most vulnerable, we all know someone who does. During Covid-19, we all knew someone we deeply cared about—a parent, grandparent, friend, spouse—who was at elevated risk. Indeed, many would likely say that, of all the fears generated by the pandemic, the greatest was not of oneself being infected but of a vulnerable loved one falling ill.

Yet it is not just during the extraordinary circumstances of a pandemic that this vulnerability exists. An older mother is vulnerable simply by living in a world that does not do enough to support the health of the aging population. A transgender husband is vulnerable because that is what it means to be gender-nonconforming in a country where 40 percent of transgender adults have reported making a suicide attempt. A Black sister-in-law is 42 percent likelier to die from breast cancer than a white woman. These vulnerabilities are a consequence of a society that has yet to fully address the structures that generate poor health and place certain groups at greater risk than others of suffering from the effects of these foundational shortcomings. Our compassion for the vulnerable in our lives must necessarily push us toward seeing how the world is currently configured to place them at a disadvantage.

In considering this vulnerability, it is important to realize that even socioeconomic advantage cannot fully ensure a healthy life. Imagine, for example, a wealthy ninety-year-old woman during the pandemic. She has all the material resources she could want. Yet for all of this, during Covid-19 she lacked the ability to do something many of us take for granted—she could not go to the grocery store herself. This was due only partly to Covid-19. As a member of a high-risk group, it made sense for the woman to avoid exposure in such a crowded place. But it was also the case that the city in which she lived was simply not designed to make it easy for older adults to navigate spaces outside their homes. As it is now, the world still largely favors the young in this respect. This may seem a moot point in her case, as she could just pay someone to shop for her. But money cannot buy the random daily encounters that happen in public spaces and give so much meaning to our lives. Humans beings are social creatures; our daily interactions are deeply supportive of our health. When we have structured our world in such a way that large segments of the population cannot fully access these interactions, we have a problem that runs deeper than the inconvenience of not being able to shop during a pandemic. It is a problem that the eyes of compassion can help us to see. Looking at the wealthy woman without compassion, it is possible to miss how this problem shapes her life. Indeed, it is easy to assume that the wealthy's material abundance covers all their needs and that our compassion is better spent on the less advantaged. But compassion insists on our common humanity; when we can see this, we can see that even a wealthy woman, at ninety, faces many of the same challenges encountered by any other woman her age of living in a society where being older is still allowed to be a significant disadvantage. She still feels the consequence of living in a world where some can be healthy but not all. Having helped us to see this, compassion then insists we do something about it. At its core, the message of compassion is that we must think about others, that the key to staying healthy lies in supporting the health of those around us. This understanding is at the heart of all the steps suggested in this book. A compassionate approach to health sees the basic fact of being human in a difficult world as the key determinant of health and disease. Because we all share this challenge, building a healthy world means creating one that maximizes the possibility of health for everyone.

Covid-19 showed us just how far we are from such a world. But it also showed us how quickly we can mobilize to fundamentally change our society at every level when we are motivated to do so. We saw many examples of compassion leading to creative thinking about how to support the health of the vulnerable. Consider the story, reported by the radio program *Here & Now*, of MJ Ryan, a Rhode Island woman who could not visit her ninety-year-old mother, Theresa, during the pandemic, due to visitor restrictions in Theresa's nursing home. Theresa suffered from dementia and heart disease, but another reason her health was declining was, in part, a lack of visitors. Her daughter's solution was to apply for a job at her mother's care facility, eventually taking a position in the laundry room. In this capacity, she was able to regularly visit with her mother, significantly improving Theresa's quality of life. MJ was also able to visit with other residents, helping to ease some of the loneliness of those days. Sadly, Theresa passed away in the fall of 2020. But that was not the end of MJ's involvement with the care facility. She informed the facility that she would be glad to come assist if needed, to support other residents. Her story is an example of how compassion can lead to actions that improve the health of populations in need. Imagine if we all practiced the active compassion of MJ Ryan, not just at the individual level but in how we structure society. In addressing her mother's isolation and how that isolation informed Theresa's poor health, MJ performed an act of both daughterly compassion and radical solidarity. She did not content herself with simply checking in with her mother over the phone or with working from a distance with her mother's caregivers to make sure she was well looked after. No, she placed herself physically at her mother's side, making a significant change in her own life and career in order to do so. It was an act both loving and courageous—she was, after all, choosing during a pandemic to work among one of the highest-risk populations. In taking this step, she modeled what compassion can do.

What might the world look like if we behaved, collectively, like MJ Ryan? It would be a world where no one would have to suffer the marginalization that creates poor health. It would mean building a society where older adults, and other groups facing isolation enforced by socioeconomic divides, are fully integrated into the wider community. It would be a world where we, as a society, have the courage to reach out, to acknowledge how connected we are, and to express solidarity and mutual concern, not judgment and stigma. Finding this courage takes compassion. It may be that, for many, this compassion first emerges with regard to our friends and loved ones. We feel compassion most strongly and immediately for those we can see, for those for whom we have long cared. The task is then to broaden this feeling, so that the scope of our compassion includes all of society.

This was the fundamental challenge of Covid-19, a challenge to which so many rose. We need to continue this work by embracing compassion as a central means of changing the world for the better, toward the goal of preventing the contagion next time. Because we do not know who will be vulnerable to the next contagion, we need to create a society that will protect us all. This will take humility—the humility to accept that certain aspects of life are out of our control. Humility also helps us to recognize all we do not know. This recognition is particularly important after Covid-19, because the pandemic was, in many ways, a validation of all we *do* know. Throughout the crisis, our scientific knowledge acquitted itself exceptionally well, as we used our understanding to develop treatments and, ultimately, a vaccine with remarkable speed. This is all the more notable when viewed in historical context. Past plagues have troubled the human species for hundreds if not thousands of years. The fact that we were able to effectively manage Covid-19, despite initial failures of prevention, within roughly a year and a half after it was first identified is a testament to our scientific knowledge and the nimbleness with which it was deployed—a success we should be proud of. Yet the scope of what we do not know remains vast. There is still much for us to learn about the large-scale forces that shape health, and we should always be mindful of the gaps in our knowledge, humble about what we do not know. These gaps informed the ways in which we stumbled during the pandemic. Even as our science moved ahead with assurance, our capacity to engage with the social, economic, and political roots of the crisis was not as surefooted.

Our ignorance relative to what we do not know is yet another reason we must have compassion for each other. We are all attempting to navigate life in the same fog—none of us know nearly enough, and it is on this foundation of incomplete knowledge that we attempt to build our lives. Given the difficulties that come with incomplete knowledge, we have a responsibility to help each other, with compassion, by building the healthiest possible world. Stigma and blame are among the mechanisms we use to avoid facing this responsibility. We need humility to transcend these forces and see clearly the roots of poor health. I will discuss humility at greater length later.

When disasters strike, they can bring out the best in us—and, at times, the worst. Experiencing a large-scale crisis is stressful, and we never quite know how we will react to such stress until we face it. One reaction is to find someone to blame. We saw many examples of this during Covid-19, with scapegoats ranging from China to the WHO to the behavior of individual Americans. The difficult truth is that disasters happen regardless of anything we do, individually or collectively. But we can take steps to limit the damage disasters can inflict, and ensure that the populations they affect are primed for resilience. We can do this by reacting to challenges with compassion and by using this compassion as the basis for building a better world. Because while it is true times of stress can lead us to treat each other poorly, it is also true that compassion can emerge from these circumstances, reminding us that the durability of our society, and our health, rests on our will-ingness to help each other in moments of challenge. At the same time, as I have argued throughout this book, we should not require the pres-sure of a disaster to motivate the actions that advance a healthier soci-ety. It is up to us to maintain the compassion that helped us through Covid-19, so that it becomes an enduring feature of our society, rather than a momentary phenomenon activated only in times of crisis. When challenges come, we have a choice to either embrace stigma and scapegoating or act with compassion. When challenges depart, the choice becomes whether or not we remember how the experience of shared threat brought out the better angels of our nature, and whether we allow them to continue guiding our actions. If we do not do so, if we do not act with compassion, then it would not be too much to say that we are the ones, collectively, who are deserving of stigma—the stigma that comes with being a society that refuses to take steps that will improve the health of all and, in particular, the health of the most vulnerable.

8

Social, Racial, and Economic Justice

Covid-19 was so all-consuming in 2020 that major events that occurred during the course of the crisis that might otherwise have been considered era-defining moments were subsumed into the larger story of the pandemic. For example, had it not been for Covid-19, the summer of 2020 might be known to history primarily as the summer John Lewis died. Lewis, who passed away that July, was a legendary American figure who spent his life working to advance the cause of justice. He was one of the original Freedom Riders—a group of activists who rode buses throughout the segregated South to challenge the racial status quo. He was also a founder of the Student Nonviolent Coordinating Committee, a key force in the struggle for civil rights. Lewis led demonstrations against racial injustice in America and helped organize the March on Washington, where Dr. Martin Luther King Jr. delivered his "I Have a Dream" speech. Lewis also delivered remarks at the march, the event's youngest speaker.

But Lewis's work for the civil rights movement went further than organizing and rhetoric. He frequently experienced violence—at sit-ins, as a Freedom Rider, and, perhaps most famously, during a march across the Edmund Pettus Bridge in Selma, Alabama, where a state trooper cracked his skull with a club, nearly killing him. His courage and tireless pursuit of a more just world eventually led to his election to the US House of Representatives, where he served for decades, representing his Georgia district. At all times during his public life, he was a touchstone for America's ongoing reckoning with racial injustice, a living reminder of the struggle and sacrifice through which a better world is slowly born.

That this process is indeed incremental, frustratingly so, was reflected by the killing of George Floyd just a few months before Lewis's death. It is painful to consider that after all the work of the civil rights movement, after all our progress toward equality before the law for people of all races, after all the distance we have traveled culturally in making racism less acceptable, it is still possible to see examples of police violence against people of color. Lewis himself said of Floyd's death and the ensuing protests:

> It made me cry to see what was happening to this person of color, but to any human being. I think it sends a message that we will not give up on justice, we will not give up on fairness, that we will continue to press, and press on for what is right, for what is fair, for what is just.

Just as Floyd's death suggested the persistence of the injustice Lewis encountered in his younger days, it also triggered events that reflected the enduring human impulse to stand against injustice, despite danger. The global protests that emerged after Floyd's death prompted a worldwide reckoning with both the challenge of racism and the challenge of security services abusing the communities they were meant to protect. The latter issue became particularly central in Nigeria, where protests emerged against the country's Special Anti-Robbery Squad, a police unit accused of abusing its power by extorting, kidnapping, torturing, and killing citizens. These protests against state-sponsored injustice were met with violence when soldiers allegedly opened fire on protesters, killing at least a dozen people.

Such violence speaks to the risk always inherent, to varying degrees, in challenging the status quo around injustice and insisting on a better world. Injustice is often so entrenched in societies that addressing it tends to mean fundamentally upsetting the established order. This can occasion pushback, and not just from those most invested in upholding an unjust status quo. A group need not directly benefit from the spoils of injustice to be hesitant about making the systemic changes necessary to end it. Civil rights activists of John Lewis's generation, for example, had to contend with both the direct physical threat of a racist power structure ruthlessly deployed against their efforts and a broader public that was not always sufficiently aware of the presence of injustice in US society. Even when this awareness was present, it did not immediately motivate the kind of actions that would make a major difference. It is one matter to get people to notice injustice; it is another to get them to care about it, and still another to get them to care enough to act to address it. Many people are conservative by nature—not necessarily in the political sense, but in the sense of not wanting to upset routines, particularly when these routines seem to support an acceptable quality of life. We are preoccupied by the daily business of living; it is all many of us can do just to attend to our responsibilities within the framework of society as it is. As long as that framework does not seem to infringe too much on our own ability to live, the notion of shifting its foundations for any reason is one we can be slow to embrace. This attitude can make the work of promoting justice challenging indeed.

This challenge is compounded by the element of physical risk that sometimes accompanies working against injustice. John Lewis and his allies faced an extreme form of this risk during the civil rights movement, as did, more recently, the protesters in Nigeria. In the United States, much of this risk centered around the danger of gathering in large groups during a pandemic. While marching during a pandemic is, of course, not the same as facing down police dogs or armed soldiers, it is indeed dangerous. The question, then, is why do movements insist on addressing injustice throughout history, even in the face of danger and resistance? The answer is that just as enduring as the human tendency among some people to accept the status quo is the refusal of others to accept any conditions that mean injustice. And while these movements of refusal can start small, history provides many examples of how they can grow to accomplish radical change.

Why is opposition to injustice such an enduring feature of our shared humanity? The answer can be seen, I would argue, in our response to Covid-19. As soon as we became aware of the threat the pandemic posed to our health, we took rapid, dramatic action to safeguard ourselves and our communities. We did so out of a visceral unease about having in our midst such an acute challenge to health. Humans, it is clear, feel a deep repugnance for what we know makes us sick. As soon as we realize something might be bad for our health, we do all we can to minimize its presence in our lives. Of course, we do not always accurately perceive what poses such a threat. As we have discussed, there remains a disconnect between what we believe represents the biggest hazards to our collective health and what is actually likeliest to sicken and kill us. Be that as it may, as soon as we decide something is a clear and present danger to health, we are willing to spare little expense of time, money, and effort in addressing it. And throughout history there have always been those who understand that injustice threatens health. In seeing this, in recognizing that injustice places health at risk, we can then find the vision and courage necessary to do what it takes to create a world without it.

And it is indeed the case that injustice is a threat to health. Throughout this book, we have discussed many examples of how poor health emerges from racial, social, and economic inequity, the root of which is fundamental injustice. This inequity is not always easy to see. Doing so means looking past our own self-interest, past our often narrow view of the world, and being open to an understanding of how others experience their lives. This is an understanding that compassion can bring. Once we have arrived at it, we can see how challenges such as racism, segregation, economic inequality, and the marginalization of communities did not just happen, that they are, in fact, consequences of injustice, rooted in history, and maintain their hold in the present day, placing health at risk. Injustice is chronic unfairness, a disadvantage that sticks. It is the product of our conscious choice to deny certain people the conditions necessary for health while allowing others to access them. Whenever we see poor health, then, it is important for us to ask ourselves if what we are seeing is actually the result of injustice.

This question is all the more necessary given the many powerful interests aligned against our asking it. Throughout history, it has served those who benefit from an unjust status quo to argue that what seems like injustice is actually the natural order of the world. This was the case, for example, with slavery in the United States, when some slave owners said that slavery was simply part of how the world was meant to be, and that it even did the slaves good to be in bondage. Given the fact that injustice is very often in the interests of the powerful, supporting their social and financial advantage, it is all the more important to be clear-eyed about injustice when it appears, with the understanding that there is nothing natural about its presence in society. Recognizing the role injustice plays in undermining health can help us identify this challenge when we encounter it, toward the goal of creating a healthier world.

Injustice falls broadly into linked but distinct categories—racial and social injustice and economic injustice. Racial and social injustice entails the disenfranchisement of a given group within culture. This can involve societal stigmas, including racism, homophobia, gender discrimination, and other means by which we disadvantage a population based on some feature of that group's identity. It can also involve a legal structure that codifies these attitudes legislatively, helping entrench modes of stigma within the network of laws that govern our lives.

For much of the country's history, for example, racial and social injustices were perpetuated at the legal level through Jim Crow laws, the political disenfranchisement of women, the denial of the right of same-sex couples to marry, and other laws or lack of legal protections that supported an unjust status quo. For this reason, promoting racial and social justice and engaging with the political process through protest, voting, and advocacy have long been synonymous. From the work of the suffragettes, who created the political conditions for the adoption of the Nineteenth Amendment, which ensured that the right to vote in the United States cannot be denied on account of sex, to the civil rights movement's strategic violation of unjust laws, advancing racial and social justice has always meant engaging with law and politics to codify equality as the rules by which we as a society organize ourselves.

It is important to note that when we talk about social injustice in the United States, of all the categories of marginalization the country has produced, its difficulties in the area of race deserve special consideration, due to race's deep entanglement with the historical and, in particular, economic roots of American society. It is for this reason that this chapter is concerned with racial injustice as an area of distinct focus. The marginalization of communities of color in the United States is of unique concern, particularly the marginalization of Black Americans. While it is true that many communities of color have suffered from deep-seated structural injustice, it is Black Americans who have, since before the country's founding, been the group most vulnerable to racial injustice. The emergence of some excellent scholarship in the past few years that has highlighted the place of anti–Blackness specifically as a detrimental force that influences health cannot, and should not, be swept up into broader generalizations around the pernicious influence of racial injustice overall. Covid-19 revealed how the institution of slavery has, over hundreds of years, continued to shape racial injustice and consequent poor health for Black Americans.

Before changes to this status quo can be achieved—before we can meaningfully mitigate the influence of slavery—movements must change public opinion around issues of injustice. One of the reasons we are so aware, to this day, of the violence perpetrated against John Lewis's generation of civil rights workers is that much of it unfolded on television. At the time, television was a new medium, and the images it broadcast had a powerful influence on the public, both in the United States and around the world. Members of the civil rights movement understood that if the world saw the brutal treatment endured by Black Americans and their allies, public opinion would likely turn against racist laws and cultural norms. This proved to be the case, as changes in the public conversation around race in the United States ultimately supported, at the political level, changes to the country's laws, changes in favor of equality and justice.

This suggests the importance of engaging with the national conversation around issues of justice, even when doing so may seem unpopular or inconvenient. Part of this engagement will involve addressing voices arguing against the necessity of systemic change. A common refrain heard by those working to end injustice is the call for patience and a tempering of seemingly radical demands. There is some wisdom, of course, in being strategic and working within existing structures to advance change. Certainly, there is no circumventing the legal and political processes that so deeply shape the reach of justice in our society, and these processes are often slow and deliberate. Yet these processes cannot be advanced toward a vision of justice without that vision first being introduced into the public conversation. This vision is almost always seen at first as radical because it is often significantly at odds with how the world operates at a given point in time. It is easy to see why the public might be wary of the disruptive potential of such a vision. But the lesson of Covid-19 is that radical disruption will occur whether we like it or not. The question is not whether we can avoid this but whether we will choose to disrupt for the sake of justice the inequities we have allowed to persist and the disasters that exploit them. The changes advocated by people such as John Lewis, changes that inform a more just world, do indeed involve letting go of the familiar, but what we are called to discard is doing us no good. By making the case that we are better off when we are a more just society, the civil rights movement was an example of how we can change our world for the healthier.

This is, of course, simplifying a complex story, one involving hardship, setbacks, and shifting cultural and political circumstances. The work of advancing social justice is the work of engaging with the fundamental forces we have been discussing in this book. As such, it means navigating often choppy waters, toward the goal of reaching a better shore. This challenge is yet another reminder of the importance of values as a guide for our endeavors—the value being, in this case, the desire for justice. It is this desire that sets social movements on a path toward engaging with a public conversation that can then shape the political process toward generating laws that support a more just world.

But the path to justice does not end with changes in public attitudes and the passage of civil rights legislation. As important as these advances are, they are not enough to ensure a fully just society. Achieving this goal takes pursuing not just social but economic justice. We have already discussed how money shapes health, and how economic advantage is unevenly distributed among populations. When we lack money, we lack the ability to be healthy, and this lack is often a result of forces beyond our individual control. These include governmental policies, the fluctuations of global financial markets, the evolution of technology, and the present-day legacy of historical circumstances. Taken together, these factors will invariably produce a measure of economic inequality, and this is not always unacceptable. Where there is economic freedom, there is always some inequality, and while this is not something to be celebrated, the twentieth century provides many examples of the abuses that can emerge from political systems that aim to enforce complete economic uniformity. Having said this, there are times when economic inequality goes beyond any tolerable level, to where it reflects fundamental injustice. The inequality that informed poor health in the United States during Covid-19, for example, was not just the inequality that emerges from the normal functioning of sensibly regulated free markets. It reflected an economy that increasingly favors the wealthiest at the expense of everyone else. It also reflected the country's history of racial injustice, which has shut many communities of color out of the opportunity to advance economically. These forces constitute conditions of economic injustice.

One symptom of this injustice was the challenge faced by front-line healthcare workers at the time of the pandemic. During Covid-19, much attention was rightly paid to these workers—to their courage and sacrifice, and to the key role they played in caring for the vulnerable and keeping society afloat at a difficult time. What this focus did not always include was an understanding of just how difficult the work of front-line care is, how Covid-19 made it exponentially harder, and how economic insecurity forced many workers to carry out their responsibilities in unsafe circumstances. This was the case for Sue Williams-Ward, a Black woman whose story was reported in October 2020 by *Kaiser Health News*. In March of that year, Williams-Ward took a job at a home healthcare agency offering $13 an hour, which for her was a $1-an-hour raise. The agency was paying a premium to attract workers after it began losing aides due to concern over pandemic safety protocols. In her new position, Williams-Ward worked with vulnerable, elderly patients, tending to their needs without the protective equipment she told her husband she had requested multiple times from her agency. She continued to work even as one of her patients showed Covid-19 symptoms. Soon Williams-Ward developed a cough. She was later hospitalized, spending weeks on a ventilator, before dying of Covid-19. In evaluating the reasons for her death, the most obvious factor is her employer's failure to provide adequate protective equipment. Perhaps less obvious, though arguably more important, were her economic circumstances. Many health workers did their jobs amid heightened risk during the pandemic because they could not afford to lose their income. That they were in this position in the first place reflects the broader challenge of economic injustice, and in particular the economic disenfranchisement of communities of color—people of color account for 62 percent of home care workers.

The intersection of race and economic disenfranchisement reflects how social and economic justice go hand in hand. It is not enough to provide legal and social equality if a country's economic engine is intractably geared toward shutting a given group out of financial—and, by implication, physical and mental—well-being. Likewise, it is not enough to ensure that everyone has access to money without also ensuring they can access the same legal protections and expectation of social equality enjoyed by everyone else. Social and economic justice are linked; there cannot be one without the other, and there cannot be health without both.

Martin Luther King Jr. well understood the link between social and economic justice. He recognized that the landmark passage of civil rights legislation was an incomplete basis for justice, that addressing racial injustice must also include addressing the economic disenfranchisement of Black Americans. In 1967, King delivered a speech titled "The Three Evils of Society" at the National Conference on New

Politics. He identified these evils as racism, economic injustice, and militarism. Leaving aside, for the purposes of this discussion, the issue of militarism—without minimizing its importance—it is worth taking a moment to consider why King identified economic injustice as equal to, and inextricable from, the social injustice of racism.

In discussing the link between poverty and the challenges faced by communities of color, King called attention to the policies underlying this disadvantage. His pointed critique of the injustices of the American economic system was informed by how this system is intertwined with the country's racial history. "We have deluded ourselves into believing the myth that capitalism grew and prospered out of the Protestant ethic of hard work and sacrifice," King said. "The fact is that capitalism was built on the exploitation and suffering of black slaves and continues to thrive on the exploitation of the poor—both black and white, both here and abroad." This statement captures the link between social and economic injustice, with the historical oppression and marginalization of Black Americans directly informing the creation of an economic system that does much to uphold inequality between races and social classes. It also insists on the role of history in shaping social and economic injustice. And it bluntly expresses how our views about individual agency can obscure our ability to see how present-day injustice is influenced by historical forces. These forces shape every aspect of our lives and societies, yet we are uncomfortable with accepting this fact, perhaps because of its implications. In the United States, we have long embraced the idea that nothing is out of reach for those who are willing to work hard, and that those who fail to achieve at the highest level have only their own lack of initiative to blame.

This is a powerful idea—and, in many ways, an empowering one. It is good to feel like we can rise by virtue of our own efforts in a society that celebrates such achievement. Yet it can also lead to the trap of thinking that anyone, or any community, that cannot rise out of socioeconomic marginalization is exclusively responsible for their predicament. This echoes the judgment and blame we sometimes direct at people who experience poor health. We feel like our society gives everyone an equal opportunity to rise or fall, and what happens to an individual is a consequence of what she has made, or failed to make, of this chance. If that person's life circumstances seem less than ideal, we are primed to assume it is because she lacked sufficient work ethic to pull herself up by her bootstraps. Perhaps even worse, this can lead to an ugly tendency to see some communities as inferior to others, which can play into racist narratives. If certain communities have consistently poorer outcomes—in employment, in social stability, in health—there is a danger the broader society will ascribe this to some inherent failing of that community, rather than to foundational forces.

The American ideal of self-reliance, then, should be regarded with a healthy amount of ambivalence. Certainly, individuals and communities bear some responsibility for their success and shortcomings, and it is true that the United States does indeed provide ample room for self-directed advancement. However, it is also true that the economic and historical forces King spoke of are deeply, even overwhelmingly, responsible for the present-day lives and health of communities. The degree to which these forces benefit some at the expense of others, basing inequality not on differences of individual merit but on systems of exploitation, is the degree to which injustice shapes the distribution of socioeconomic disadvantage and poor health. When our national narrative prevents us from seeing this, it ceases to be empowering, becoming instead a negative influence on the health of the population.

The first step toward promoting justice, then, is being able to see where it is lacking, even when doing so is uncomfortable or necessitates a reevaluation of key narratives. Sometimes this injustice is—or should be—obvious to all, as with the killing of George Floyd. Other times, incomplete understanding of the roots of injustice can make it harder to see. This can be complicated by the fact that some simply do not wish to see injustice, either because they are the beneficiaries of the status quo or because accepting the presence of widespread injustice is simply too painful, its implications too profound. Recognizing injustice forces a reckoning with the fact that we are not perfect, that we may actually be deeply flawed. Awareness of these flaws leads to the difficult, necessary work of addressing them, and to the fundamental changes this implies. For these reasons, when we are confronted with a stark fact about America's racial divide—for example, how the burden of Covid-19 fell disproportionately on communities of color—there are many incentives to look the other way, to find explanations that do not involve injustice. These explanations may even entail some truth. We may look at the gaps in Black-white mortality during Covid-19, for example, and choose to see primarily a challenge of pure economics, with the material disadvantage faced by many communities of color driving their poor health. The challenge with this analysis is when it stops there, when we do not ask why the communities faced this disadvantage in the first place. To do so would be to confront a legacy of injustice, originating with the crime of slavery, that extends into the present day. It would be to face the hard truth of our history, a history we would perhaps rather not see.

Our hesitance to take this step is a key barrier standing between the world as it is and a more just world, a world fully supportive of health. It is also understandable. Self-reflection is difficult, particularly when it leads to truths we would prefer to avoid. Yet if we avoid these truths, our efforts to build a healthier world will always come up short. One way of facing them is through a thought experiment, conceived by the philosopher John Rawls. The experiment invites us to design a new society. It can be anything—it can be a democracy or a dictatorship; it can be broadly equal, or home to rigid hierarchies. The only catch to our freedom in shaping this world is that once we have designed it, we must live in it—and we are not allowed to know in advance what place in the society we will occupy. If we design a society with slavery, there is as much a chance we will be a slave as there is we will be a slave owner. If we design a world characterized by injustice, there is no guarantee we will not bear the brunt of it ourselves. We simply cannot know. Rawls called this lack of knowing the veil of ignorance.

When considering our society in the real world, we should always be asking ourselves: Is this the world we would design from behind the veil of ignorance? Is it truly just, or are we only able to think it so because we occupy a privileged place in society? These are hard questions that bring us into contact with the ways in which we still tolerate injustice. They force us to think about how certain groups suffer poorer health than others due to the circumstances of their lives, circumstances that they did not themselves create. For example, the fact that a Black baby in the United States is likelier to have a shorter, sicker life than a white baby is not a consequence of anything that baby did, nor of anything her parents did. It is a consequence of the foundational forces that began shaping health in the United States long before the child or her parents were born. If anyone is responsible for how these forces aligned, it is those who were present at the very start of the United States who did not need to concern themselves with having to live without the full privileges available at their time, and who acquiesced in the creation of foundational injustices that echo in the present.

The founders of this country had a unique opportunity to come as close as it may be possible to get to applying Rawls's thought experiment to the real world, designing a nation almost from scratch. Unfortunately, they did not do so from behind the veil of ignorance. The country they made was shaped largely by the interests of the powerful at the expense of the marginalized. The founders created a society that was, at least in the beginning, most aligned with the interests of property-owning white men. It is true that they also built into the foundations of this society ideals of equality that, though not fully realized at the time, have served as an aspiration pulling us toward a more just society. Yet it is important not to forget how those who initially advanced these ideals did not necessarily mean for them to be applied to everyone. From the start, our country's ideals have been a paradox, simultaneously advancing justice and serving as ideological cover for some of the worst injustices human beings can inflict on each other.

The United States is, of course, not unique in this regard. History provides many examples of countries built on foundational injustices. As time passes, societies are able to reach a point where the privileged can convince themselves that these injustices do not even exist, and that those who say they do are trying to evade taking responsibility for their own lives. The irony here is that this represents what is arguably an even greater evasion than that committed by an individual shirking personal responsibility for his problems. It is the evasion of collective responsibility for our failures as a society.

This speaks to a key point about health and the forces that shape it. It reflects how health intersects with narrative, with the stories we tell ourselves. At present, the mainstream version of this story is largely a tale of doctors, pharmaceuticals, and the power of treatment to cure us when we are sick. It is not so much a story of the social, economic, environmental, and political forces that shape health, nor has it sufficiently captured the role of justice in influencing these conditions. Our story, then, needs to change, if we are to create a world that supports health.

In a sense, our vision of health is much like our vision of our country. A country is more than a government and borders, more than a network of laws and physical infrastructure. It is a story a group of people share about who they are. Such stories are informed by culture, collective values, and aspirations. The difficulty arises when we confuse the aspirational quality of our story—who we wish to be—with the reality of who we are. This confusion can cause us to turn a blind eye to injustice when we assume that all the necessary battles on behalf of justice have been won and our present condition is one of complete fulfillment of our national promise.

The United States, for example, was founded on an ideal of freedom, one we have not entirely fulfilled. However, not all Americans have accepted that we have fallen short of our aspirations. Many still insist that the playing field is level for all, despite the inequities that persist in this country, inequities that became particularly clear during Covid-19. What is perhaps ironic about this is that even at the time of our country's founding, many were aware of how we were betraying our core ideals. This was even clear to those who personally wrote those ideals into our founding documents. Thomas Jefferson, the founding figure arguably most responsible for the ideals of liberty enshrined in the Declaration of Independence, famously contradicted the values he set down in that document through his ownership of slaves. What is perhaps less well known is the extent to which he was himself conscious of this hypocrisy and its implications for the nation he helped found. He fully understood the injustice in his country's midst, even as he helped perpetuate it. Of slavery, he once wrote:

> I can say with conscious truth that there is not a man on earth who would sacrifice more than I would, to relieve us from this heavy reproach, in any <u>practicable</u> way. The cession of that kind of property, for so it is misnamed, is a bagatelle which would not cost me a second thought, if, in that way, a general emancipation and <u>expatriation</u> could be effected: and, gradually, and with due sacrifices, I think it might be. But, as it is, we have the wolf by the ear, and we can neither hold him, nor safely let him go. Justice is in one scale, and self-preservation in the other.

He was not alone in his understanding of the evil of slavery. Abigail Adams, for her part, hated slavery, fully recognizing it as an injustice. She was also aware of another key injustice of that time—the exclusion of women from full political and social rights. This awareness prompted her to advocate on behalf of women, as it did others at the time, including Jefferson's vice president, Aaron Burr, who believed in complete equality between women and men.

It is important to raise these examples to show that even in the days when our national narrative was first being constructed, there were figures living who saw the injustices threatening to undermine its promise of liberty. And they recognized injustice not only as a marked contradiction of the national project but also as a potentially destabilizing influence on society. It is good to be reminded that it is always possible to see injustice clearly, even when doing so is at odds with prevailing present-day attitudes. We often hear that we must not apply modern judgments to the study of historical figures who lived in times when certain injustices were accepted as a matter of course. Yet the examples of Adams, Burr, and Jefferson reflect how it is possible to recognize injustice even when doing so places us against the grain of public opinion and our own material interests or forces us to acknowledge the ways we might be hypocritical as a society. If this could be the case nearly 250 years ago, it is inexcusable for us to turn a blind eye to injustice in the present, whether that injustice emerges from the legacy of past inequity, as in the case of racism in the United States, or takes a form that is entirely new.

However, it is also important not to forget just how accepted even the most egregious injustices long were throughout history, and the degree to which this acceptance depended on the willingness of societies to do nothing about them. It is a sad fact that while all individuals have the capacity to commit crimes and acts of injustice, it takes whole populations to commit the largest-scale offenses. While it is true that many spoke out against slavery, for example, it is also true that slavery existed on this continent for hundreds of years because far more people actively participated in this evil, or at least declined to try to stop it. They did not act against this injustice because they either did not see it as wrong or recognized it for what it was but still did not speak out. It is worth asking ourselves what injustices we currently tolerate that future generations may look back on with the same question for us that we have for the generations that tolerated slavery: "What were they *thinking?*"

I would argue that the health inequities exposed and exploited by Covid-19 will be high on the list of injustices that prompt this question. It is not that these inequities rival slavery in their poisonous effect on society, however much they are informed by its legacy. It is that we allow them to persist despite all our wealth, knowledge, and mostly good intentions. It is the fact that the *Chicago Sun-Times* had cause to run a story in November 2020 about anxiety among some members of the Black community about taking a Covid-19 vaccine due to their distrust of the government and health authorities. "We've been hood-winked so many times with vaccines," said the Rev. Floyd James, the pastor of Greater Rock Missionary Baptist Church in North Lawndale, Chicago. "We've been experimented on by the government, by the scientific community and the hospitals." This sentiment is understand-able given how deeply entrenched the legacy of racial injustice is in the United States, a legacy that has indeed been perpetuated by key institutions, from government to public health. Perhaps the most infa-mous example of this was the Tuskegee Study, where the US Public Health Service told the study participants, a group of low-income Black men with syphilis, that they were receiving treatment for their "bad blood," when, in fact, treatment was withheld so that the dis-ease's progression could be studied. That such an injustice might have been condoned by anyone—let alone by those in positions of federal or scientific authority—speaks to the depth of the injustice that has long characterized our society and undermined our health. It is this injustice that kept our health so vulnerable for so long, right up until catastrophe struck during Covid-19 and we found ourselves lost at sea. It is what made the deaths of George Floyd and John Lewis so reso-nant in occurring so near each other. Their proximity was a reminder to the nation of the shame of still facing the same injustices that first motivated Lewis to join a movement for social and economic justice. It is the shame of important business left unfinished.

Such unfinished business is not, of course, unique to the United States. Globally, we face significant injustices, the persistence of which will likely look no more explicable to future generations than our acceptance of health inequities in this country. Chief among them is an issue that will do much to decide whether there will, in fact, be future generations at all: the challenge of climate change. Climate change exists at the intersection of social and economic injustice. It reflects economics by emerging as it does from systems of global indus-trialization that have generated the pollution that currently threatens the planet. It reflects inequities within society by disproportionately harming low-resource parts of the world, places that have contrib-uted much less to the problem than the richer, more industrialized nations that have so far escaped its worst effects. Our continued fail-ure to adequately address climate change is an example of the human capability of turning a blind eye to injustice even when the problem could not be clearer. Climate change represents how continued injustice can threaten to destabilize whole societies—though in the case of the climate crisis the threat extends beyond even society itself, to challenge the very ecosystem on which we depend for our survival. If we wonder how past generations could have countenanced deep and obvious injustice in their midst, we need only look to climate change for an example of how such errors can repeat themselves.

The reason for this recurrence of historical error was well summarized by Jefferson: "Justice is in one scale, and self-preservation in the other." We behave as if ignoring the roots of injustice will allow us to preserve a status quo that works well for everyone. At the same time, those for whom the status quo works best—the powerful—may see, in overlooking or even further entrenching injustice, a means of preserving their own privilege. But all are mistaken in these actions. We can no more ignore injustice and expect to sustain well-being than we can ignore cracks in the foundation of a house and expect it to remain upright. Because the injustices embedded in the status quo do not, in fact, support a healthy society for anyone. As we have discussed throughout this book, as long as any population is exposed to the conditions that create poor health, everyone's health is at risk. This recalls the words of Dr. King: "Injustice anywhere is a threat to justice everywhere." The cycles of history, the recurrence of the same injustice generation after generation, can make it seem as though injustice is a problem without a solution, as though it is an unfortunate fact of life we simply must live with. Fortunately, we have the example of people such as Dr. King and John Lewis to show that this impression is false, that we can indeed stand against injustice. Taking this stand requires an honest view of our collective flaws and the courage to make significant, even disruptive changes to achieve a society without injustice. In doing so, we need not neglect our instinct for self-preservation—on the contrary, creating such a society is the best step we can take toward creating a more sustainable shared context. Covid-19 showed us that a world that tolerates injustice places limits on its capacity to be healthy. Once we have seen injustice, we have a responsibility to not look away, to fix the racial, social, and economic inequities that generate poor health.

9

Health as a Public Good

When we think about health, we typically think about individuals rather than whole societies. It is not difficult to see why. Our earliest frame of reference for health is our own body—our own experience of sickness and recovery, of visits to the doctor and of taking the drugs she prescribed. It can be as difficult to view health from outside this frame of reference as it is to see the world from beyond the perspective of our individual subjectivity. It takes work, compassion, and practical understanding of the interconnectedness of health to move beyond our early view of health as an individual concern and to see health as it is: something of collective importance, upheld by collective support.

Covid-19 necessitated this more expansive understanding of health. During the pandemic, it was difficult to see health as anything other than interconnected. It was a time when even the healthiest individuals faced a viral threat that leveraged the links between people in order to spread and cause harm. In this context, it did not matter very much what we as individuals might have done throughout our lives to stay healthy. Certainly, a baseline of good health, supported by good habits, was not unhelpful in the face of the virus, but the most overwhelming influence on health at the time of Covid-19 was the virus itself and the conditions that shaped its spread. Addressing these conditions meant thinking of health not as an individual concern but as a public good.

Public goods are resources that benefit everyone and are supported by common investment. They include parks, the public school system, national security, the environment—anything we have come to regard as too important to be accessible exclusively to those who can pay. An example of a public good is fire safety. In our society, we have accepted that fire safety is too crucial to our collective well-being to be left to the market. However, this was not always the case. The work of fire-fighting traces its history back to the Roman era. The first Roman fire brigade was started by Marcus Licinius Crassus, a general and political figure of great wealth. His skill in accumulating this wealth was evident in his approach to firefighting. If a house caught fire, representatives of Crassus would arrive with an offer to buy it from its present owner. This offer would be made while the place was still burning. If the offer was accepted, Crassus's fire brigade would put out the blaze, but if it was refused, the house was left to burn. Such a practice is almost a par-ody of cutthroat capitalism — the precise opposite of the pursuit of the public good. In writing about it for the *New Yorker*, Hendrik Hertzberg described this approach to getting money as "a manner strikingly like the operations of health-insurance companies a couple of millennia later." The comparison is apt, given how the evolution of firefighting over the years reflects how attitudes can shift from seeing something as a private commodity to seeing it as a public good, with implications for our attitudes toward health.

As we know from our present approach to firefighting, the privat-ized Roman model did not remain the dominant means of addressing fire safety in communities. Today, we have decided that fire safety is too important to depend on individuals' capacity to pay for it, so we fund it as a public good. What is more, we have embraced fire preven-tion as a means of reducing the need for firefighting. In the United States, starting roughly after the outbreak of the Great Chicago Fire in the nineteenth century, fire departments have moved toward a model of helping communities adopt strategies to reduce the occurrence of fires. This has entailed the creation of safer houses and the promo-tion of a culture of prevention based on best practices in fire safety. A far cry from the predatory capitalism of Crassus, this approach to fire prevention is based on investing in fire safety as a public good. This investment has indeed succeeded in preventing fires. In 1977, there were 5,865 civilian deaths that occurred as a result of home fires in the United States. In 2016, there were 2,735.

It is significant that the evolution of firefighting from a private commodity to a public good has overlapped with the evolution of fire safety from a purely reactive endeavor to a preventive one. Investment in fire safety is ultimately investment in health, and health is funda-mentally about avoiding disease and injury, not simply treating it when

it strikes. Investing in health as a public good requires collective investment in creating the conditions for health to flourish. In the area of
fire safety, this means creating a context where fires are less likely to
occur. Looking at what it takes to create this context shows us a microcosm of all we have been discussing in this book. This includes engaging with politics to pass laws that aid fire prevention, working within
culture to create healthier norms, and shaping the built environment
so that the places where we live, work, and play are more resistant to
fires. All these actions have been guided by the understanding that a
world where fires are less likely benefits everybody, so the work of
creating this world ought to be supported by our collective effort. That
is why we have come together to engage with foundational forces to
make this world a reality.

Unfortunately, fire prevention is just one part of the much larger
project of building a world that is fully healthy, a task we have not
always performed well. While we have achieved steady success in
reducing the danger of home fires, Covid-19 exposed our shortcomings in reducing poor health, shortcomings exacerbated by our treatment of health as a commodity rather than as something we can all
share. Humans have a stubborn tendency to magnify the illusion of
separation between individuals and groups and to minimize the reality of how closely linked we actually are. That this tendency has long
been with us is reflected by the actions of Crassus. He clearly did not
consider the possibility that letting houses burn could lead to a fire
spreading throughout the city, threatening everyone's life and property,
including his own. That this risk would not have occurred to him, or,
if it did, that he ignored it in his pursuit of profit, suggests how easy it
is for us to find ways to insist on our separation from each other, even
when the reality of our connection is clear. This insistence helps keep
us from seeing health as a public good.

We saw this during Covid-19 when it came to the issue of masks.
One of the key reasons it was so difficult to convince people to wear
masks at the time of the pandemic, in addition to President Trump's
willingness to make the issue into political theater, was that the very
idea of making a collective sacrifice in order to improve our health was
alien to us. The extent of our alienation from this idea was revealed by
the relative slightness of what was being asked of us during Covid-19.
There is nothing particularly onerous about wearing a mask—it is
barely a sacrifice at all. Yet many in the United States reacted to what

they were being asked to do as if King George III himself had come back to life to levy a new round of taxation without representation. We may run the risk in this country of being too close to this behavior to realize how strange and counterproductive it truly is. It is particularly strange that we should be more hostile to even the mildest notion of collective sacrifice than we are to a system that permits something as fundamental as health to be treated as a mere commodity.

In the United States, our capacity to see health as a public good is complicated by this individualistic streak, which keeps the spirit of Crassus alive in our approach to the forces that generate health. During Covid-19, this spirit was reflected in the actions of one of the few people alive with wealth comparable to that of the famous Roman: Tesla CEO Elon Musk. The billionaire and business magnate made news for downplaying the severity of the pandemic and for resisting the lockdowns, even in the pandemic's particularly uncertain early months. At one point, he tweeted to his millions of Twitter followers, "Tesla is restarting production today against Alameda County rules. I will be on the line with everyone else. If anyone is arrested, I ask that it only be me." Earlier in the pandemic, he was particularly blunt in his attitude toward the lockdown, tweeting, "FREE AMERICA NOW."

Musk has a reputation as a maverick innovator, yet in expressing these sentiments, he was projecting an attitude that is, in the United States, deeply conventional. It is an attitude that prioritizes the idea of individual liberty above all, with the added, uniquely American twist of conflating individual liberty with the ability of powerful corporations to do whatever they want. Absent from this outlook is any notion of the public good. Musk's intense focus on his business may help drive his innovation, but it misses the broader importance of health as a necessary condition for not just the smooth functioning of business but the long-term sustainability of society. If everyone in a society is sick, it will not matter if factories have the latitude to remain open in a pandemic. The productive power of a given company or individual will not generate an immunity to poor health. It is possible to believe that exceptional energy or talent can create special categories for people and organizations that justify holding them to a different standard than others, letting them opt out of the framework of rules within which the rest of us must live, a framework that supports health. In the United States particularly, we are receptive to the spirit of Shakespeare's line "[N]ice customs curtsy to great kings." We celebrate those whose individual initiative seems to set them apart from others, and we often cheer them when they bend the rules in pursuit of their goals. Yet even the exceptional are not excepted from the interconnectedness of health. The same links that connect your health to mine and my health to yours connect us to the health of Elon Musk, his employees, and everyone else with whom we share the world. That no one is exempt from this network was reflected by Musk's own brush with Covid-19. In the fall of 2020, he confirmed that he had been infected with the virus; fortunately, his case was not severe and he soon recovered. His experience of the disease, like that of President Trump and others working at the highest levels of government, reflects how power and privilege cannot make anyone any less a part of the basic interconnectedness of our shared existence.

In many ways, Covid-19 was a clarifying moment. It showed the extent to which an individualistic, go-our-own-way streak—easily romanticized and quintessentially American though it may be—does absolutely nothing to keep us healthy. It is difficult to overstate how little good this mentality did during Covid-19. In the face of mass sickness and death, with the failure of our society to adequately safeguard health laid bare, protestations of individual liberty did nothing but postpone our collective embrace of the only philosophy that can actually prevent disease on a large scale: the embrace of health as a public good. I am emphasizing this point because in the United States we have long listened to those who raise the cry of individual liberty above all even when that cry leads to nothing but preventable injury and disease—even when the choice is literally between liberty and death. At the same time, efforts to address health as a public good are vulnerable to accusations of paternalism or are vilified as an attempted power grab by sinister, faceless bureaucrats. It is striking how common such paranoia and conspiracy thinking were even during Covid-19, when the need for a concerted effort to support health was at its most acute. The anti-vaccine movement, for example, was quite active at that time, particularly online, where memes and misinformation casting doubt on the safety and efficacy of vaccines were in robust supply. These conspiracies also suggested something was not right about the timing of the vaccine. Because the story announcing an effective Covid-19 vaccine broke not long after the US election was called for Joe Biden, some in conservative circles suggested coordination between vaccine developers, the media, and the Democratic Party to delay the announcement to hurt the political prospects of President Trump and help those of Biden. This reflects the extent to which conspiratorial thinking during Covid-19 was likely informed by the context of a heated presidential election, with partisans on both the left and the right often wary that the outcome might be subverted by bad-faith actors within government and media. Even controlling for this historically unique moment, the mistrust of institutional efforts to address Covid-19 reflected something long-standing about our society's approach to health. This mistrust has undermined our capacity to approach health as a public good while fueling a hostility to the very entities through which this approach might be pursued.

Engaging with health as a public good, then, means making the case against entrenched, individualistic hostility to the collective work of building a better society. It should be unacceptable that the idea of rational, restrained paternalism should be more frowned on than an approach to civic life that maximizes the freedom to sicken and die in an ever-expanding range of ways while narrowing our options for living healthfully. It is also important to note that actions often characterized as paternalism tend to be broadly supportive of health. They represent an effort to use societal institutions to create a context that supports our collective well-being, steps informed by a concern for the public good. Turning away from this approach during the pandemic left society at the mercy of its most irresponsible members, prolonging one of the most difficult periods in our country's history for the sake of a shallow interpretation of our core ideals, one that does us little good in the best of times and functions as a form of suicide in the worst. It is on us to move beyond this way of thinking, recognizing the harm it has done, if we are to create space for a new engagement with health, one informed by our common responsibility to care for each other's well-being.

It is perhaps understandable that we have been slow to see health as a public good. The links connecting our health, and the importance of an approach to health shaped by an awareness of these links, can seem abstract, particularly compared to vivid appeals to individual liberty. It is only really able to remain abstract, however, when times are relatively stable. In the absence of acute crisis, the argument that our well-being depends entirely on maximizing individual liberty, while still wrong, is less obviously false. At such times, our society remains characterized by health haves and have-nots, but the conditions are in place for the haves to fail to see the have-nots clearly, and for them to be able to believe that the presence of societal disadvantage does not in any way threaten their own well-being. It is when crisis comes that the limits of this outlook become apparent. Health as a public good is fundamentally an abstract idea only until a challenge such as a virus makes inescapable the links that bind our health together. In normal times, the average person may feel worlds apart from someone like Elon Musk. In the time of Covid-19, however, the conditions of a pandemic made it clear that, in fact, our health is intimately linked, connecting the wealthiest with the most disadvantaged in a way that is tangible, quantifiable.

These links are well illustrated by Figure 9.1. A visualization of the Covid-19 transmission chain, it shows how individuals served as focal points for virus transmission within broader networks. It is striking to see these networks presented in this way, with each individual linked to an ever-unfolding number of associations. It is particularly help-ful to see how even one additional interaction links to many others, reflecting how important it was during the pandemic to limit our daily

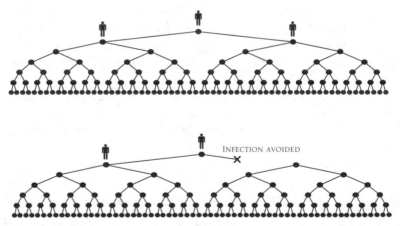

CORONAVIRUS CHAIN OF TRANSMISSION WITHOUT AND WITH LIMITING SOCIAL CONTACTS

INFECTION AVOIDED

Figure 9.1. Adapted from figure found at The Learning Network. What's Going On in This Graph? | Coronavirus Protective Measures. *The New York Times.* March 26, 2020. https://www.nytimes.com/2020/03/26/learning/ whats-going-on-in-this-graph-coronavirus-protective-measures.html. Accessed January 4, 2021.

interactions in order to minimize the spread of the disease. While it may still have been possible for some people to avoid thinking about the interconnectedness of health, it was not possible for anyone to escape its practical effects.

There are few better arguments for treating health as a public good than an awareness of how interconnected our health truly is. When one ceases to think "My health is in *my* hands" and starts to think "My health is in *our* hands," one has found an outlook upon which a healthy society can be based. Thinking of health this way is by no means intuitive. That is why it can be so easy, even during a pandemic, to feel that our choices about risk and exposure are solely personal, concerning no one but ourselves. Yet Figure 9.1 clearly indicates how our actions are embedded within a web of connection.

The pandemic had the effect of cutting through the abstraction that can characterize our thinking about the networks that shape health, giving us a clearer sense of the connection that links us all. We experienced this connection at the personal level, through navigating quarantine. Anyone living in a household with multiple people at the time of the pandemic understood that it was not enough to choose, as individuals, to make responsible decisions. To maximize safety, the entire household needed to treat health as a public good—as something to be shared by everyone, and which could be maintained only through collective support. This meant that everyone living in a given place needed to think carefully about how their individual actions might affect the health of everyone else.

The importance of this thinking was reflected, on a larger scale, by the eightieth annual Sturgis Motorcycle Rally, held in Sturgis, South Dakota. The rally attracts about a half million motorcycle enthusiasts each year, who come from across the country to take part in the event. The 2020 rally happened in August of that year and was notable for its flouting of Covid-19 protocols: there was little mask-wearing or physical distancing, and the whole event was infused with the individualistic spirit typified by biker culture. All this resulted in what may have been one of the most significant superspreader events of the pandemic. Research estimates there were more than 260,000 Covid-19 cases linked to the rally. These cases were dispersed throughout the country as rallygoers returned home from the event, carrying the contagion with them. This spread illustrates the connections that inform our health, and how no amount of rugged individualism can change the fact that we are part of this web.

As the weeks and months of the pandemic progressed, our thinking about how to stay healthy started to include more than choices about whether or not to wear a mask, eventually leading to an engagement with the full range of conditions necessary for sustaining health. Nutritious food, education, opportunities to exercise, leisure time, and financial stability are all examples of these conditions, and as the pandemic wore on, we came to see just how necessary they are for health. During that time, we often heard of how "pandemic fatigue" was causing some people to ease their adherence to the lockdown, as they chose to accept the risk of taking trips, gathering with friends, and other activities that may not have been strictly necessary for survival but which many nevertheless found painful to give up for an extended period of time. Some saw these lapses as irresponsibility, or simply exhaustion winning out. I would argue, however, that they reflected the reality of health: that health is more than the absence of disease, that it also depends on goods such as access to quality schooling, socializing with family and friends, and spaces where it is possible to regularly exercise. The pandemic offered us a chance to pursue health as exclusively the avoidance of contagion—all we had to do to greatly minimize risk was give up all the other goods that make life meaningful. The fact that so many people were unwilling or unable to make this sacrifice reflects the importance of these factors in shaping a truly healthy life.

As we came to understand this during the pandemic, we started to make efforts at the household level to pursue health as a public good by working to ensure that those with whom we were living could access the resources necessary for health. Parents worked to make sure their kids could retain some sense of normalcy in their education; roommates shared the responsibility of ordering and picking up nutritious food so households would have more than canned goods and processed fare to eat; we all learned to prioritize the upkeep of common outdoor spaces such as parks where communities could exercise while keeping a distance. In short, we recognized that health is a public good, and we worked to support it by broadening access to the non-medical resources that make it possible. This was not so much a choice on our part as it was a natural alignment with the reality of health. For many, there was no other way to sustainably live for the better part of a year under pandemic conditions. In more stable times, it is indeed possible to feel one can go it alone, living each day without an awareness of how much every one of us depends on others. Typically, it is only the sudden occurrence of hardship or tragedy that brings the stubborn individualist face-to-face with this reality of connection. She feels she can take care of herself—until the day comes when she cannot, when the challenges of life make it necessary to ask for help. Some people are able to postpone this day for a long time, but no one can forever avoid it.

Before Covid-19, our country was engaged in this evasion, ducking the truth of our common existence. The pandemic was the day we thought we could avoid, the day when reality asserted itself and we were placed in a position where it was no longer possible to pretend the human condition is somehow optional. It was time, finally, to ask for help—and to give it. In supporting each other through Covid-19, we were able to see how asking for help is not a matter of weakness or lack of self-sufficiency, that at the core of giving and receiving assistance is the understanding that we all find ourselves on both sides of this dynamic at various points in life. In giving help today, we recognize that tomorrow we might be the ones in need of support. This recognition is at the core of what it means to prioritize the public good. When we cannot see past the individual, we are liable to miss this reciprocity, seeing only how we are called to give help to others and overlooking how we might one day need it ourselves. Sadly, for some this is cause for resentment and a feeling of being taken advantage of by those who may not "deserve" aid. What is missing is the shared sense that we could all be the ones needing help at some point. When we realize, say, that our house could burn tomorrow, we are likelier to invest in fire prevention today, as a means of self-preservation. It would be nice, of course, if no one needed an answer to the question "What's in it for me?" before investing in the public good, but there is indeed an answer for those who ask. That answer is: "Everything. Your health, your children's health, and the long-term stability of society on which we all depend." One can therefore be as self-interested as Crassus and still have ample cause for investing in the public good.

In addition to clarifying the importance of this investment, the pandemic made it easy to see the limits of our current approach. Throughout the experience of Covid-19, we hoped for an end to the crisis not just because we feared catching the virus but also because we desired a better quality of life. Deprived of the physical presence of friends and family, threatened by job loss and financial insecurity, and confined largely to our homes, we saw how key such contextual factors are to health. We may have been able to avoid Covid-19, but simply avoiding the virus was not enough to make us feel healthy. Perhaps it was for a little while, but in the long run we needed more. Likewise, living in a society where we can treat many diseases can, at the point of cure, create the short-term illusion of health. But if we are cured simply to return to lives that unfold in a context that is not conducive to well-being, then we have embraced this illusion at the expense of creating a world that can keep us truly healthy.

We have now seen the cost of failing to create such a world. The pandemic presented many examples of how our failure to pursue health as a public good has become unsustainable. One of the key features of the pandemic was how, at various points, a rise in cases threatened to overwhelm the healthcare system in the United States. The fall of 2020 was a particularly difficult time for the pandemic. By then, the country had been struggling with Covid-19 for more than half a year, leading many to become tired of Covid-19 restrictions at what turned out to be the worst possible time. This fatigue, combined with cold weather causing more indoor gatherings and the holidays bringing people together, led cases to surge in the United States. This rise in cases caused many hospitals to report staff shortages. The challenge was particularly acute for rural hospitals. Many lacked staff and resources before the crisis, and the emergence of Covid-19 threatened to fray this already threadbare system even further. Often, rural hospitals simply did not have space to accommodate the surge in Covid-19 patients, and so needed to find beds for them elsewhere. In November 2020, *USA Today* reported on the challenges faced by these hospitals. Matthew Shahan, CEO of West River Health Services in Hettinger, North Dakota, was quoted as saying that before the pandemic, "I don't think I ever made a call to another hospital, administrator to administrator, begging them to take a patient." Yet the crisis required his staff to reach out to multiple hospitals asking if space was available for critically ill patients. Indeed, the situation became so dire in North Dakota that the governor even announced that healthcare workers with asymptomatic cases of the virus could continue working with Covid-19 patients in hospitals.

In a *Fast Company* article, "What Doctors at Overwhelmed Rural Hospitals Are Facing, in Their Own Words," Jennifer Bacani McKenney, a doctor from Fredonia, Kansas, wrote, "The community is tired, frustrated, and stubborn. Politicians talk about relying on personal responsibility to end the pandemic, but I don't see a majority of people wearing masks in public spaces despite pleas from health professionals. Some people are scared. Others act as if Covid-19 doesn't exist." Her words capture how failure to treat health as a public good—as our collective responsibility—creates the conditions for the burden of supporting health to fall disproportionately on the shoulders of healthcare providers.

The influx of patients during Covid-19 reflects an approach to health that focuses on medicine alone. We think that doctors and treatments are all we need to stay healthy, but this is not the case. When the pandemic struck the United States, it was met by a healthcare workforce that comprised some of the most intelligent and courageous people our society produces. These workers had at their disposal cutting-edge technology and the support of communities who regarded them, rightly, as heroes. When the second wave of Covid-19 hit, they even had the benefit of months' worth of experience dealing with the disease, giving them a far better sense of how to address the virus than in the pandemic's early days. Yet around the country, healthcare systems were still overwhelmed. This was not the fault of our drugs or our technology, and it certainly was not the fault of the medical teams. It was the fault of an approach to health that prizes medicine above all. When we do not see health as a public good, when we narrowly restrict the areas where we engage with health to doctors' offices and hospitals, we make it all but inevitable that our healthcare system will be overwhelmed in the event of a crisis on the scale of Covid-19.

In my role as dean of the Boston University School of Public Health, I often have the chance to deliver presentations about how we can best create a world that generates health. In these presentations, I frequently use the metaphor of a soccer game to describe our approach to health. Preventing disease is like preventing a soccer ball from entering your team's goal. The goalie represents the healthcare system—doctors and medicines. The rest of the team represents all the other forces we have been discussing in this book: money, politics, power, place, and so on. Anyone who knows about soccer knows that the aim of a good team is to ensure that the ball never reaches the goalie. Ideally, the team should be skilled enough that the goalie serves only as the last line of defense. If the goalie is medicine, the rest of the team represents our engagement with the broader forces that shape health. By pursuing this engagement, we can help ensure that the ball only rarely reaches the goalie. A healthy society is one where the goalie could be absent for the whole game and her team would still win because the rest of the team is playing so well that the ball never has a chance to get near her net.

This is precisely the opposite of the state of play when Covid-19 struck. For the metaphor to properly reflect the conditions of the pandemic, the goalie's teammates would have to be largely incapacitated, to the point where the other team's players could line up just a few feet from the goal and spend the game kicking the ball directly at the net. Under these circumstances, a team could employ the greatest goalie the world has ever seen and that team would still lose badly. It would not take a diehard soccer fan to recognize such a match as ludicrously one-sided and to question the wisdom of a team even playing at all in such a sorry state. Yet the state of this team was more or less the state of our approach to health in the United States when Covid-19 emerged. And it will remain the state of our approach to health if we do not learn the lessons of the pandemic and start treating health like a public good.

When we treat health as a public good, we acknowledge the importance not just of the rest of the soccer team but of the factor that is most important in carrying the group to victory: teamwork. The first principle of teamwork is placing collective interests over those of the individual, in pursuit of the common good. This is not to say that the individual does not matter, only that she understands her interests are best served by a shared focus on a vision of success. In sports, success means working together to win the game. In creating a healthy society, it means engaging with nonmedical factors that influence health and shaping them toward a vision of a healthier world. This is possible only when we approach health with a spirit of common purpose, embracing the perspective that it is a public good. Our individualistic approach to health is unsustainable, its weakness made clear by the pandemic. By evading our common responsibility for health, we created an undue burden for our healthcare workers, one that, for all their skill and commitment, they found difficult to manage.

We need a new model, one where we ease this burden by sharing it as a society, and we should not wait for the next crisis to strike before adopting this fresh approach. Fortunately, just as our individualist approach to health is rooted in our shared national values, there is much in the American philosophy to inform a pursuit of health as a public good. From the Progressive Era to the New Deal to the Great Society, the United States has long seen ambitious initiatives advanced in the name of the public good. These programs represent an evolution in our collective understanding of what constitutes the public good and how it can best be supported at the national level. We first articulated our approach to public goods in the preamble to the US Constitution, which reads:

> We the People of the United States, in Order to form a more perfect Union, establish Justice, insure domestic Tranquility, provide for the common defense, promote the general Welfare, and secure the Blessings of Liberty to ourselves and our Posterity, do ordain and establish this Constitution for the United States of America.

In this brief statement, the Constitution defined the country's legal framework as a means of supporting the public good. It specifically defines the establishment of justice and the provision of the common defense as fit areas for national engagement. Yet it also leaves room for the expansion of this rather narrow definition of the public good. Having named promoting "the general welfare" as an object for common national endeavor, the Constitution implies the importance of working together as a country in pursuit of this goal. In the years since the document was written, we have decided that the general welfare means far more than the founders likely intended. Yet we have hesitated to commit to expanding this definition to include the pursuit of health. We have hesitated in large part because we feel that our health is sufficiently supported by medicine, and all that is necessary for a healthy society is to broaden access to doctors and treatments. Not only is this untrue, but it risks us seeing health the way Crassus saw fire safety: as something to be bought and sold.

The truth is, we cannot buy health for ourselves. What we can buy is healthcare, and that can only help us after we are already sick. At the individual level, this approach means we will always be in danger of poor health. At the collective level, it means accepting a permanent reservoir of preventable disease and death within society, the presence of health haves and have-nots, and, when crisis strikes, an overwhelmed healthcare system. These are the real-world effects of choosing to go it alone when it comes to health. Could there be anything worse for the general welfare? Or to ask another question: do we want an approach to health that takes care of us when we are sick, or one that prevents us from getting sick to begin with? Certainly, the two approaches are not mutually exclusive. But we are currently so disproportionately invested in treatment that this focus comes at the expense of engaging with health as a public good.

While this overreliance on medicine is a key reason for our hesitance to embrace health as a public good, it is not, I suspect, the only reason. There is also how engaging with health as a public good would inform our understanding of our collective responsibility to each other. It would imply we have a duty to address health at the structural level, so that everyone can live a healthy life, regardless of identity or social status. It would call on us to place health at the core of all we do, from policymaking to industry to urban planning. Pursuing health as a public good nationally would also open the door to making this pursuit a global priority. To do so would be to assume a significant responsibility, one that calls on us to make big changes to how we live our lives and organize our society. It is understandable that we might balk at such a heavy lift. Yet this is a responsibility we cannot shirk if we are to prevent the contagion next time.

Perhaps most fundamentally, pursuing health as a public good means acknowledging health is a human right. There must be no degrees of privilege when it comes to accessing the conditions that support health. We cannot be healthy unless everyone is healthy. This means we need to take steps to support the health of the vulnerable, because their vulnerability is our vulnerability—and in supporting their right to health, we are supporting our own. To do this, we have to create the proper conditions, engaging with the foundational forces that shape health. Our capacity for this engagement rests on our willingness to see health as a public good, something that is supported by collective investment.

Finally, it is important to acknowledge that pursuing health as a public good will require trade-offs. Centrally, this pursuit requires that we let go of our overwhelming focus on medicine. Covid-19 revealed that the idea that treatment alone can safeguard our health is an illusion. However, it is a comforting illusion, and what comforts us can be difficult to give up. It would indeed be nice to think that medicine is all we need to create a healthy society. There is an appealing simplicity to the idea that preventing disease is just a matter of purchasing the right pills and keeping our medical appointments. But experience tells us that this is a limited approach, dangerously so. It is putting all the pressure on our goalie and ignoring the rest of the players on the field. Instead, we need to invest in building the best possible team, guided by the same spirit of collective endeavor that supports success in any undertaking that requires effective collaboration.

Once we have embraced this spirit, we can apply it to the kind of ambitious initiatives that truly shape a healthier world. We can do this by building on the steps we took during Covid-19 to safeguard health at the social, economic, and political levels, with an eye toward preventing disease before it can take hold. When we understand that health is a human right rather than a private commodity, it follows that we invest in making sure it is accessible to everyone. The question we must ask is: is health worth this investment? Before the pandemic, most people would have answered yes; after, our yes should be unanimous. While we were ultimately able to navigate the pandemic, few would say our performance during Covid-19 was optimal. How might we have done if we had indeed pursued health as a public good before the crisis struck? Imagine, for a moment, that our commitment to supporting our collective health had meant that we had invested in a Marshall Plan for health. That we chose for even one year to spend the amount we typically invest in medicine on the pursuit of social and racial justice within communities, on the construction of healthier living spaces, and on a more robust social safety net. Had Covid-19 emerged in such a world, it would have been far less likely to cause the harm it did. Investing in the creation of this society is akin to investing in fire prevention, creating a context where a spark cannot become a blaze. The first step toward this is the recognition that health is a public good.

SECTION 4

A Science for a Better Health

I O

Understanding What
Matters Most

So far in this book, I have been making the case for engagement
with the nonmedical forces that shape health. I have maintained
this focus for two reasons. First, because these forces are the central
determinants of health. They are what determine whether or not we
are a healthy society, and they shape our vulnerability in the face of
infectious disease. We cannot prevent the contagion next time without engaging with these forces. Second, because these forces currently
do not command enough attention in our conversation about health,
particularly relative to their importance, and even more particularly
compared to the overwhelming focus we put on medicine.

In the interest of helping to correct this imbalance, I realize that this
book may read at times more like a text about sociology, political science, economics, or even architecture than as a book about the science
of health, skewed as that science often is toward treatment. This refo-
cusing is, I think, necessary to inform a conversation that helps create a
healthier world. However, it should not obscure the role of science in
bringing that world about. Just because we have not discussed the science of developing treatments—such as the vaccines that did so much
to end the Covid-19 crisis—does not mean that science is not integral
to creating a context where contagion cannot take hold. Indeed, it is
science that helps us to understand the link between health and the
forces we have discussed so far. The work of my field, academic public
health, is the work of applying scientific methodology to the pursuit
of this understanding. This science has helped us to see, for example,
the links between economics and specific health outcomes, the role
of social networks in safeguarding mental health, how the legacy of

slavery has shaped mortality in certain geographic areas, and the relationship between politics, government policies, and population health. In bringing us these data, science helps generate the knowledge that lets us chart a better course for health, so we can steer our ship in the right direction.

For these reasons, promoting a science for better health is core to creating a healthier world, post-Covid-19. I will close this book, then, with a section on the pursuit of this science, and how science can inform the steps we need to take toward better health for all. I will start with a discussion of how science can shape our understanding of what matters most for health.

As we have seen throughout this book, the forces that shape health are complex. It can be difficult to draw from this complexity a clear path forward for actions we must take to get us, collectively, to better health. This is, in part, why we focus so intensely on medicine—because elevating the role of medicine makes the work of promoting health appear simple. When we focus on medicine, it seems clear what matters most: creating better drugs and ensuring that as many people as possible can access them. When we set aside this simple portrayal in favor of the more complex picture of what supporting health really entails, science can help us to understand this complexity. It can help us to see that if we want to be healthy, we must engage with the complex ways in which foundational forces interact to shape the context of our daily lives.

Covid-19 highlighted the importance of understanding this complexity. It also reflected just how difficult it can be to maintain focus on what matters most, particularly in the midst of a crisis. Given this difficulty, it is always worth returning to first principles, to what is most fundamental about our health. So, even if we feel we already know, it is worth asking again: what mattered most during Covid-19?

In hindsight, after a pandemic, with effective treatments well in hand, it can seem like medicine was obviously the most important factor. And indeed, the extraordinary success of vaccine development, in record time, is what brought this pandemic to an end. Yet we all know that this is complicated by the anxiety many of us feel—or, at least, should feel—about our continued vulnerability to contagion. We are able to vaccinate against the coronavirus, but only against a specific coronavirus. The Covid-19 vaccine will not prevent a new virus from emerging. Medicine can protect us from diseases, but it cannot protect us from disease itself.

This was clear even at the height of the pandemic, with the pursuit of a vaccine reinforcing our pro-treatment narrative to an unprecedented degree. Even then, the messy complexity of the forces that really shape health was difficult to ignore. This was the case, for example, in conversations about who should receive the vaccine first. In early December 2020, the Advisory Committee on Immunization Practices (ACIP) met to discuss this issue. The ACIP operates within the CDC to provide guidance on addressing vaccine-preventable diseases in the United States. In their December meeting, they voted 13 to 1 to advise that healthcare workers and people staffing and living in long-term care facilities be the first to receive the vaccine. That the ACIP voted so overwhelmingly this way reflects the importance of the nonmedical forces that shape health. If all that mattered was the development of a vaccine, if socioeconomic conditions were not a factor in shaping Covid-19 risk, it would hardly matter who received the vaccine first. Yet socioeconomic factors had, by that point, made clear that certain populations were indeed at greater risk, and this risk was most acute for healthcare workers and people in long-term care facilities. The reason for this risk had to do with the nature of the virus, yes, but also with circumstances of employment, economics, and race. Throughout the pandemic, science played a key role in helping us understand the link between these conditions and Covid-19 risk, so when it came time to make important choices, such as who gets the vaccine first, we were able to do so guided by a sense of what matters most.

This was no small feat. It is not always easy to understand what matters most. The interplay of factors that generate health can obscure what is most important, misdirect our efforts, and lead us down blind alleys. This is particularly the case when we face an unprecedented crisis.

During Covid-19, I spent much quarantine time listening to podcasts about world history. Hearing accounts of wars, revolutions, the rise of social movements, and the general churn of incidents that is our past, I was struck by how much disagreement there is among historians about what mattered most in creating the conditions for key events. What, for example, mattered most in causing the French Revolution? Was it economic frustration? Poor leadership on the part of the king? Social and philosophical movements of the era? Going further back, what was the central cause of the fall of the Roman Empire? Historians have had centuries to address these questions and still have not been able to identify a consensus response. Compare this to the challenge of understanding what matters most for health, and attempting to do so amid complexity, doubt, the evolving circumstances of a pandemic, and the knowledge that failure could result in choices that place thousands, if not millions, of lives at risk. In this context, it is uniquely important to have sound data and a core awareness of the foundational forces that shape health.

As I have already suggested, our performance during Covid-19 is probably best characterized as "muddling through." We did much right, but certainly not everything, and not nearly enough to serve us well in the event of a new, potentially worse contagion. It is important to be honest about our performance if we are to take the necessary steps to do better next time. Sometimes we acted in accordance with what mattered most; sometimes we did not. Few would say we acted perfectly, but it is worth pointing out the complete failure we managed to avoid, and what that failure could have looked like. Visualizing this failure is a useful exercise, both as a means of benchmarking our current state of public health preparedness and as a way of motivating improvement. A total failure to fully integrate what matters most into our approach to health could have looked like a level of societal collapse we have not yet seen in the United States. Specifically, it could recall *The Raft of the Medusa*, a nineteenth-century painting by Théodore Géricault (Figure 10.1).

The painting depicts a variation of the central metaphor of this book: a ship. The image was inspired by the true story of the *Méduse*, a French Royal Navy frigate that was wrecked off the coast of Senegal in 1816. It had been more than two decades since the captain of the ship had last sailed, and he had received his commission due to political favoritism rather than ability—his chief qualification was that he happened to be a monarchist, placing him in good standing with the leaders of the time. His incompetence and poor navigation were blamed for the ship running aground on a sandbank. After it became clear the ship could not be freed and that there were not enough lifeboats for everyone, about 150 passengers and crew boarded a raft they had constructed and departed on a thirteen-day journey of starvation, death, and cannibalism that left only fifteen people alive, five of whom died shortly after they were rescued. The painting depicts a frenzied scene,

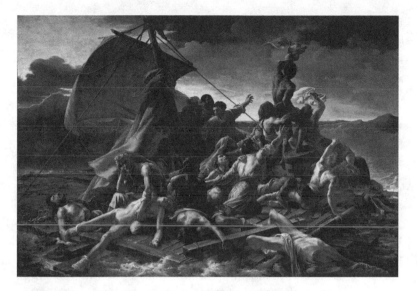

Figure 10.1. Géricault T. *The Raft of the Medusa*. 1819. The Louvre Museum. Paris, France. Copied from Wikimedia Commons website https://commons .wikimedia.org/wiki/File:JEAN_LOUIS_THEODORE_GÉRICAULT_ -_La_Balsa_de_la_Medusa_(Museo_del_Louvre,_1818-19).jpg. Accessed January 4, 2021. Public domain.

as desperate survivors mingle with corpses and attempt to catch the attention of a distant ship as it sails away. Géricault had done extensive research in preparation for the work, interviewing survivors and visiting morgues to practice his depiction of dead bodies. The result is a harrowing vision of suffering and societal breakdown.

The painting made a significant impression when it was unveiled. Some found the striking scene compelling; others were repelled by both its style and content. All of these responses were valid. The painting is powerful enough to stop viewers in their tracks and make them consider what could have caused the tragedy captured by the image. The causes of the disaster are familiar to our discussion in this book: they are political (the politics that elevated an incompetent to a position of command) and they are a fundamental misjudgment of the proper course to take (in this case, leading the ship to ruin).

The sheer extremity of the event depicted in the painting is a reminder of how the misalignment of large-scale forces can produce

deep human tragedy. What is perhaps most disturbing about what happened to the *Méduse* was the relative banality of the mistakes that led
to the wreck. When we think of horrors like those suffered by the
people on that raft, it is easier to imagine they are somehow the result
of evil intent than it is to think they could emerge from mere political
failure and incompetence. But the truth is that these are precisely the
conditions that can produce some of the most acute suffering humans
experience, and they arise when we lose sight of what matters most.

This was a painful lesson of Covid-19. Who might have predicted,
in the years leading up to the pandemic, that we were setting the stage
for some of the worst suffering this country has seen? Certainly, we
could see there were areas of dysfunction in our society, caused by
our unwillingness to address the foundational forces that shape health.
Perhaps we even understood how these conditions were generating
preventable disease and mortality. But millions of cases of infectious
disease? Hundreds of thousands of deaths? Widespread economic dev-
astation? Surely such outcomes could not be the result of the same
conditions about which we may have felt a vague sense of disapproval
or unease but none of the fear that acute threats would typically evoke.
Yet these are indeed the conditions that led to the disaster we all
experienced.

Just as *The Raft of the Medusa* provides a powerful portrait of how
conditions and institutional failures can create a context for suffering
and poor health, the pandemic provided many stories that reflect a
similar dynamic. I have already shared a number of these stories, and
could well share many more to underlie this point. However, to illustrate these forces at work and how they reflect what matters most
for health, I will here take a page from Géricault's book and paint a
heightened portrait of one such story. The depiction is fictional, but
it conveys, I think, the truth of how the experience of Covid-19 was
shaped by larger forces. The utility of a fictional portrait is that it allows
us to glimpse inner motivations and speculate about how a real-world
event may have intersected with the hopes, fears, and deepest values
of individuals. This perspective can help inform our understanding of
what matters most.

Imagine a woman named Jean. She is about thirty years old and lives
in a small town in West Virginia, where she was raised. Her upbringing
was not marked by privilege. For generations, her town had been a
mining community, where digging for coal provided stable jobs that

paid well. When Jean was a child, however, the mine closed, devastating the community and leading to widespread unemployment. Jean's father had been a miner, and the loss of work made him bitter. He turned to alcohol and was often physically abusive to Jean, her mother, and her two sisters.

One of the few bright spots of Jean's formative years was her involvement with her church. Churchgoing was common where she grew up, and it was a rare Sunday when much of the town was not to be found in pews. Going to church was simply what one did in the community. In addition to providing spiritual sustenance, it was a place to see friends and family, to hear music, and to momentarily transcend the hardships of life. For Jean, going to church was the highlight of her week, and always had been, even when she was a child. While some kids resist going to church, she had always been eager to get there. She would sit and listen with rapt attention during the sermon, memorizing the preacher's words, which she would deliver to her stuffed animals when she returned home. The message of church—of the sermons, of the people gathered together in harmony—allowed her to glimpse a vision of life she did not often see in her own family. It was a vision of compassion and mutual care, driven by the notion that, despite the difficulties of life, the force behind everything was fundamentally good, and could be accessed through faith and common purpose.

To live with such a belief is, of course, to have it regularly tested. The basic condition of life is one of challenge, and the Covid-19 crisis represented a significant one. When the scope of the pandemic became clear, the crisis seemed to Jean like something out of the Bible—like one of the plagues of Egypt, or like the tribulations sent to afflict Job. It felt even more like a judgment in seeming to particularly target certain groups. Jean's community was hit hard. There had always been a lot of poor health among the people of her town—addiction, obesity, and other chronic conditions worsened through lack of the health insurance that mining jobs once provided. The pandemic exploited these challenges to create a situation that did indeed recall something more akin to ancient tales of plague than anything the community had yet seen, even in its lean years of socioeconomic marginalization.

Through it all, Jean continued going to church. She was not alone. Despite the threat of infection, her community still filled the pews each Sunday. Some wore masks, some did not. All seemed to feel that the pandemic called for expressions of faith—in God and in the community spirit in which they saw God reflected. As the months of Covid-19 continued, it became clear that the community was not doing enough through mask-wearing and physical distancing to stop the spread of the virus, and the regular church services were likely worsening the situation. However, the community kept attending, and Jean kept going with them.

This story is fictional, but it is very much a composite of many true stories that unfolded during the pandemic. There was, for example, the group of people who attended a California religious service on Mother's Day 2020. It was later revealed that one of the roughly 180 attendees had been infected with Covid-19. While it is difficult to know definitively how the service affected the spread of the virus, cases in the surrounding county doubled in the two weeks after Mother's Day, though only one of the cases was definitively linked to the service. Then there was a case in Sacramento County, where seventy-one people linked to a single church were found to be infected. It would be easy to be glibly moralistic about these cases, to feel, if not outright say, that these people had no one but themselves to blame for making the dangerous choice to congregate in the midst of a pandemic. But this impulse would be wrong. We have already discussed how scapegoating people for their poor health is counterproductive and reflects an inaccurate view of where health truly comes from. We can only choose to be as healthy as our context allows us to be. So what looks like a simple choice—say, whether or not to go to church—is, in fact, embedded within layers of complexity.

I told the story of Jean in an effort to unpack some of this complexity. Her habit of churchgoing was a product of both her cultural context and her individual zeal. Her zeal was in part a response to her home life and the cruelty of her father. Her father's behavior was both his choice and a particularly negative reaction to his economic circumstances. Those economic circumstances were shaped by trends in the mining industry and the broader economic forces that influenced them. At a perhaps deeper level, Jean's choice to go to church was shaped by her values; it was a personal response to the human condition, and similar responses have influenced religious belief since time immemorial. Then, of course, there was the emergence of a historic pandemic, which made the decision to regularly attend church into something deeply consequential for health.

During Covid-19, when we heard about people like Jean, people who risked infection by attending church services, we were likely to think that what mattered most for their health was the choice to risk going to a public gathering. What we would likely not have done was unfold a hypothetical story in our heads like the one I just told about Jean, one showing how a person's choice to go to church in a pandemic could be an act so consistent with her belief structure and socioeconomic context that it might not even occur to her as being a choice at all. Given the power of context to shape behavior, what matters most is the interplay of forces that shape the lives of individuals and communities.

Just as Jean's experience of the pandemic, and the experiences of individuals like her, was shaped by this interplay of forces, so was our collective experience of Covid-19. Jean's deeply personal response to Covid-19 and the choices she made during the pandemic were informed by what she felt mattered most in her life. These priorities were linked to everything she experienced and to the larger forces that made this experience what it was. Likewise, our collective choices about Covid-19 were informed by the interplay of culture, politics, geography, economic trends, and other such factors, which shaped our priorities, the choices that emerged from those priorities, and, ultimately, our health.

These choices were broadly encouraging, as they often showed us to be willing to take dramatic action on behalf of health. They were also a snapshot of our understanding of what matters most for health, and how this understanding does not always align with the reality of what makes us healthy. The most significant story of 2020 may well be not so much the virus itself as our response to it. The distinction is a fine but necessary one, shedding much light on how we understand what matters most. During the pandemic, we made a clear choice to sacrifice societal functioning in the name of doing all we could to stop the short-term spread of poor health. This meant accepting a measure of severe economic distress, job loss, and a disrupted education for millions of children. The last point is profoundly significant for long-term health in the United States.

I am occasionally asked what intervention I would select to improve health in this country if I could only choose one. My answer is always universal investment in early childhood education. A good education is one of the best assets a person can receive to help ensure a healthy life. It is linked with increased life expectancy, healthier decision-making, and less sickness. The earlier a child is given access to quality education, the better. While many teachers rose to the challenge of providing quality remote learning to students during the pandemic, it is nevertheless true that many students simply learn better in the classroom, with the in-person support the school setting provides. During the pandemic, the data were clear that schools were not high-risk areas for virus transmission. Despite these data, concern over the possibility of spread in schools was strong enough that many local governments faced pushback when trying to reopen schools, even in a limited capacity. This meant that many children experienced sustained educational disruption at an age when such influences can shape the lifelong trajectory of health.

The argument for making this sacrifice, as well as for the economic sacrifices of the lockdown, is "We did what we had to do to safeguard health." This mentality is understandable—yet it is also, to an extent, misguided. In doing what we thought we had to do for health, we were neglecting the factors that matter most to preventing disease. Early in the pandemic, when we knew little about the nature of the disease or how it would affect populations, it made sense for us to embrace a widespread lockdown. As bad as Covid-19 was, there was a moment when, for all we knew, it could have been far worse. In that moment, a lockdown was the best tool at our disposal for mitigating the short-term effects of this unknown threat. The cost of this was to temporarily deprioritize the broader forces that shape health. We accepted the socioeconomic disruption we knew a lockdown would cause in order to forestall the worst-case pandemic scenario. At that time, under those specific circumstances, this was indeed acting in accordance with what mattered most.

But these conditions of relative ignorance about Covid-19 would not last long. As the pandemic progressed, science gave us a clearer sense of the disease—whom it affected, how it spread, and what steps could best help to reduce transmission. We learned, for example, that the key points of transmission were unventilated indoor spaces where many people gathered. We also learned that certain groups were at greater risk of the disease than others, and that while young and healthy people still sickened and died from Covid-19, the greater risk, by far, was to people with preexisting conditions and those over the age of sixty-five. And we saw how the spread of the pandemic linked to the broader forces that shape health, how it was likelier to transmit among the socioeconomically marginalized. It is significant that the communities most at risk of Covid-19 were those for whom the effects of the lockdown—namely, economic instability and lack of access to quality education—were long-standing challenges, predating the pandemic. This reflected a situation where, with the lockdown, we chose to pause our engagement with the factors that matter most for our long-term health while we learned more about the virus—only to find that our vulnerability to the disease had been most deeply shaped by these very factors.

As we learned more about Covid-19, we changed much of our behavior to align with updates to our knowledge. Early in the pandemic, for example, we did not yet know the extent to which the virus could survive on surfaces. This led to an embrace of disinfectant wipes, as we used them to clean doorknobs, countertops, and even groceries. Despite this early embrace, there is a reason that masks remain an enduring symbol of the pandemic and wipes largely do not. This is because as the pandemic wore on, our scientific inquiries into the nature of the virus showed us that the disease transmits mainly through airborne droplets and that the risk of catching it from surfaces is very small. So the practice of wiping down groceries faded, and we no longer placed as much emphasis on the importance of disinfecting surfaces, even as we maintained an emphasis on other best practices. Guided by science, we kept our focus on what mattered most.

But why did we embrace this shift in focus? Why did we not continue to emphasize the need to disinfect groceries, even though the risk of transmission via surfaces was small? Is it not true that small risk is not the same as no risk? Why do we need to emphasize what matters most to health when we could just emphasize everything, big and small, that matters to health, for the sake of caution and thoroughness? These are important questions. The answer is that health requires trade-offs. We have only so much energy and only so many resources. To be healthy, we need to make choices about where we apply our focus, or we risk undermining our efforts.

We saw this dynamic unfold during the pandemic. Early in the pandemic, health authorities made significant requests of the population, asking millions to dramatically alter their behavior in the name of health. People complied because they understood how critical taking these steps was to safeguarding health—their own health and that of their community. But this did not make complying with these requests easy. The trade-off of setting aside normal life for an indefinite period of time depended on being able to trust that those calling for the sacrifice were doing so guided by the best possible data, aligning their advice with what matters most for health. With this in mind, health authorities had a responsibility to listen to these data, to ensure that they did not ask the population to waste energy and focus on steps that were peripheral to the core mission of staying healthy at a particularly difficult time. Anything less would be both a betrayal of trust and counterproductive to the work of generating support for the measures that protect health. Simply put: it does not do to cry wolf. When the public has confidence that it is being asked to behave in accordance with the science of health, it is far likelier to comply than if it feels recommendations are being made arbitrarily, without regard for what actually matters most.

During the pandemic, there were many examples of how public trust was undermined by the perception that leaders were not making choices guided by what matters most. At one point, a viral tweet circulated featuring a video of Los Angeles restaurant owner Angela Marsden emotionally denouncing Los Angeles mayor Eric Garcetti and California governor Gavin Newsom for what she characterized as their hypocrisy on outdoor dining bans. She said her outdoor dining space had been shut down, but just across the street from her restaurant a movie studio had been allowed to set up a large outdoor dining tent. "I'm losing everything. Everything I own is being taken away from me and they set up a movie company right next to my outdoor patio, which is right over here," she said. "And people wonder why I'm protesting and why I have had enough."

Her anger reflects what can happen when it seems like we have lost collective focus on what matters most. It is one thing when it is clear we are all being asked to make sacrifices that the science clearly shows will help safeguard health. It is another thing entirely when the manner in which these sacrifices are being called for suggests they may not actually reflect the reality of the threat. By shutting down restaurants but seeming to hold movie studios to a different standard, it was possible to think the lockdown was not actually a public health necessity if it could be so easily set aside for the powerful and privileged. Given the fact that the burden of lockdowns did indeed fall most heavily on the vulnerable—such as small businesses, retail workers, and individuals who could not telecommute—it was all the more important for those restrictions to be implemented in an evenhanded way, and only for as long as they were absolutely necessary in the face of an immediate, potentially catastrophic threat. As the pandemic wore on and we learned more about the disease, it became clearer that keeping in place the lockdown measures we adopted at the start of the crisis no longer aligned with what mattered most. At the same time, inconsistent and at times unfair implementation of the lockdown resulted in the justified sense that such policies were actually making the situation far worse for the vulnerable whose livelihoods they threatened, even as the privileged were able to suffer less from the policies they themselves imposed.

At the time of the pandemic, I was part of a research team that analyzed the lockdown's effect on public health. We found that lockdowns and socially restrictive policies can undermine health in both the short and long terms, creating particular challenges for vulnerable populations. Our work suggested that the harmful consequences of such policies should be considered in decision-making about pandemic response. These policies can cause harm for all the reasons we have been discussing in this book—by affecting the socioeconomic context in which we live in ways that threaten health. We know this because there are robust data on how health and disease link to this context. It became something of a political flashpoint to make this observation during the pandemic. Given the polarization of opinion about Covid-19, particularly in the United States, it was not uncommon to see pro-lockdown attitudes characterized as liberal opinion and an anti-lockdown attitude characterized as a conservative view. Yet the science painted a more nuanced picture. Lockdowns were indeed necessary in the beginning, but as the pandemic unfolded, it became apparent that the socioeconomic costs of the pandemic mattered at least as much as the threat of the virus, and the importance of those socioeconomic factors only grew as Covid-19 continued. It is also true that while many understood this, our decisions about Covid-19 mitigation did not always reflect the reality of what mattered most. The fact that this was at times clearer to the general public than it was to key decision-makers reflects why, if we are to avoid such misalignment in the face of future pandemics, it is necessary for us to better understand, at every level of society, what matters most for health.

To return for a moment to Jean: In choosing to go to church during a pandemic, Jean was, from a certain point of view, acting in defiance of what matters most for health, if what matters most is being physically distant from contagious disease. However, when her decision is viewed in the full context of her life, we can see how it aligned with factors of core importance to her well-being. Church, for Jean, was a hub of community and emotional uplift, helping to create social cohesion even as economic trends threatened to fracture her community and undermine its health. Throughout the pandemic, we saw churches play this role, helping to sustain communities in ways that may have seemed inexplicable to those who viewed supporting health during the pandemic entirely through the lens of whether or not communities chose to physically isolate. In December 2020, *Kaiser Health News* reported on how, for example, Black churches were helping congregants navigate the overlapping challenges of Covid-19, racial injustice, and health inequities. One of the stories featured was that of Wilma Mayfield, whose place of worship, Lincoln Memorial Baptist Church in Durham, North Carolina, invited a psychologist to deliver a virtual presentation about mental health during Covid-19 and how the challenge of the moment was disproportionately affecting communities of color. The presentation also included practical steps on how to improve mental health during the stress of Covid-19. "They said to get up and get out," Mayfield said. "So I did." She said the presentation "opened up doors" for her, as she took the speaker's advice to be more active as a means of improving mental health.

The emergence of churches as spaces where communities could come together during the pandemic to find this kind of support represents a gesture toward the factors that truly matter most for health. These factors are, collectively, the context in which our lives unfold—the socioeconomic forces that ultimately do more to shape our health than any virus, even one as significant as Covid-19. In our understandable rush to address the immediate threat of the virus, we occasionally lost sight of these factors, just as we tend to lose sight of them in our focus on medicine. During the pandemic, our early push to avoid contagion was slow to pivot to a broader engagement with the forces that matter most for health. This was partly due to lack of clear communication about what the science said about how to best address the disease—waters muddied by often incoherent messaging at the federal level—and partly due to our entrenched belief that staying healthy is simply a matter of doctors and pharmaceuticals and treatments rather than of the forces we have been discussing throughout this book.

It is not too late to make the necessary pivot toward engaging with what matters most for health. It is, in fact, more important than ever that we prioritize these factors, if we are to prevent the contagion next time. The social, political, and economic dimensions of health are just as core to health between pandemics as they are when such challenges strike. Indeed, they are what allow outbreaks to become global crises in the first place, if they are not handled properly and well in advance. So we should handle them in advance, learning the lessons of Covid-19. This will take continued scientific engagement with the forces that matter most for health. The spectacular success of vaccine development during the pandemic will raise the understandable temptation of redoubling focus on medicine, orienting even more of our scientific energies toward treatments. We should take care that this does not distract us from robust exploration of the socioeconomic forces that shape health.

There was much research done during the pandemic, some of which I have cited in this book, that examined how these forces intersected with the crisis to shape health. This represents an important area for long-term study—the socioeconomic disruptions caused by the pandemic will continue to influence health for years, if not generations, to come. By continuing to trace this influence, we can help keep focus on what matters most to health. The fact that during the pandemic the immediate threat of the virus was regarded by some as greater than the threat of long-term socioeconomic instability reflects how far we have to go to cultivate a full understanding of what matters most to health. At the same time, the fact that many of us still were willing to accept calculated risks during the pandemic to attend church, send our kids to school, and take other actions motivated by a wish to access the socioeconomic resources necessary for health reflects that we indeed understand, on a deep level, what matters most for health. At the moment, this understanding exists as a kind of collective cognitive dissonance, as our focus and investment still overwhelmingly skew away from these foundational factors. Preventing the contagion next time will depend in large part on our ability to align this focus with what matters most, so we can take steps guided by the right priorities, not waiting until crisis strikes to engage with these core issues.

11

Working in Complexity and Doubt

In late 2020, Covid-19 cases were surging across the United States. In Oklahoma, for example, the state had seen 233,336 cases and 2,042 deaths by early December. However, there was one part of Oklahoma that was in a far better position—that was, in fact, a model of how to best address the crisis. In a challenging context, the Cherokee Nation had found a way to keep cases and death rates within its borders relatively low, even as the crisis raged in the surrounding area. It did so through a number of key choices made at the beginning of the pandemic. These included embracing an early mask mandate—instituted in spring 2020—and taking proactive steps to learn about best practices for dealing with the disease. At the start of the pandemic, when the CDC had not yet released guidance on contact tracing, Lisa Pivec, senior director of public health for Cherokee Nation Health Services, looked up the WHO's work responding to Ebola to learn about the protocols for tracing. The Cherokee Nation took additional steps, including providing free drive-through testing, protecting vulnerable older adults, safeguarding food security, stockpiling personal protective equipment (PPE), and holding regular Covid-19 task force meetings.

These measures paid off. By the time Usha Lee McFarling reported on the Cherokee Nation's performance for *STAT News* in November 2020, the nation had reopened Sequoyah High School for fall in-person learning and largely resumed elective dental and medical procedures. These actions were supported by relatively low case rates, particularly when compared to other tribal areas. In summer 2020, the CDC reported that as a whole, American Indian and Alaskan Native populations had Covid-19 case rates 3.5 times higher than the white population. The Navajo Nation, with about 170,000 citizens, had suffered about 13,000 cases and 602 deaths. By contrast, the Cherokee Nation reported a bit over 4,000 cases and 33 deaths out of its roughly 140,000 citizens. This contrast was likely shaped by the differences in resources and response between the two nations. In its reporting, *STAT News* noted at the time that in the Navajo Nation, "Covid testing, PPE, and sometimes even running water are in short supply."

Given the high case rate in the surrounding community and challenges faced by other Indigenous groups, it is clear that the Cherokee Nation's comprehensive approach to the pandemic, shaped by key early decision-making, made a significant and likely decisive difference in improving the health outcomes of that community. Its surefooted choices at the start of the pandemic are all the more noteworthy for having been made in a context of complexity and doubt. The start of the pandemic was a uniquely difficult moment. It was when we knew the least, yet when our decisions arguably mattered the most. The Cherokee Nation navigated this moment by seeking out best practices, guided by past examples, then taking what seemed to be the most effective steps for dealing with the disease. In such contexts, with high stakes and limited information, there is a temptation to either make gut decisions, based entirely on what feels right rather than on the facts, or to become paralyzed by the lack of information and wait until more data come in. The Cherokee Nation struck an admirable balance, acting on the data they had while not letting the lack of complete information cause them to miss the window of opportunity to take commonsense steps, laying the foundations for an effective long-term response.

Unfortunately, not everyone engaged with the start of the pandemic the same way as the Cherokee Nation. The state of Oklahoma itself, for example, was slow to embrace many of the measures that the Cherokee Nation took in the pandemic's early days. As late as September 2020, the state's governor, Kevin Stitt, declined to issue a statewide mask mandate, saying he believed one to be "unenforceable," though he did support individual cities in Oklahoma issuing the mandates. He said, "We think that's a local decision and I'm not going to mandate that statewide because I don't think there's a one size fits all approach to this virus." His approach to mask mandates is noteworthy because it reflects the kind of decisions that can emerge from contexts of complexity and doubt. There is an element of equivocation to such an approach, of choosing to take one path but also leaving the door slightly open to taking another. We are familiar with such decisions, as we all tend to make them. It is human nature to hedge when making choices in the face of life's complexity. We like to give ourselves an "out" whenever possible, and most of the time there is nothing terribly wrong with doing so. However, in the context of a health crisis, when lives depend on navigating complexity to arrive at clear, effective choices, such an approach can be counterproductive, even catastrophic.

This chapter is about how, when we are faced with complexity and doubt, we can make decisions about health that align with the approach of the Cherokee Nation and avoid some of the mistakes made by other leadership teams during Covid-19. Working in complexity and doubt requires, above all, balance. On one hand, we must be able to identify what we do know and respect the science enough to integrate this information into the choices we make. On the other hand, we must appreciate the limits of our understanding while not being paralyzed by them. We must cultivate a comfort with ambiguity and doubt, so that we can position ourselves to make decisions that support health.

During Covid-19, we made a number of choices. They include, but are not limited to, closing schools and businesses; embracing, to the extent we could, a stay-at-home culture; telecommuting whenever possible to avoid workplace exposures; and generally adhering to a lockdown that, however unevenly applied, amounted to a yearlong closure of society as we have long known it. We paused nonessential travel, as daily commutes and holiday trips became a risky proposition. We also embraced mask-wearing—patchily, grudgingly, but in the end more or less collectively.

In thinking about these choices, it is also worth considering the path we chose not to take. This starts with our choice of how we thought about the pandemic. On the scale of the common cold to the Black Death, when all is said and done, we chose to think of Covid-19 as a threat somewhere in the mid- to lower range of this scale. It did not always seem like this, of course. Our response to Covid-19, with its sense of turning the world upside down, certainly could appear in the moment as though we were treating the disease as a true civilization-threatening plague. Yet there were no Flagellants roaming the streets. Quarantine did not involve literally locking the infected in their homes. There was no painting red crosses on the doors of the infected to indicate the presence of disease, as was done during the Black Death. And while there was scapegoating and societal tension, far more widespread were the compassion and mutual concern that played such a fundamental role in helping us navigate the crisis.

We also chose not to underreact. Just as we did not treat Covid-19 like the Black Death, we also did not treat it like the flu. We could have, of course. The human capacity for denial is immense. Families deny for years the existence of painful secrets and deep rifts. Individuals deny failings and vulnerabilities. Societies deny monstrous injustices in their midst. In this context, denying the true nature of a disease is a comparatively minor matter. When faced with Covid-19, we could have simply ignored the data about its risks and the disproportionate danger it posed to certain populations and carried on as if everything was basically fine. Indeed, many people chose this path, pretending as if the virus was overblown or even a hoax. But these people, vocal as many of them were, remained a minority throughout the pandemic. The majority treated Covid-19 with the seriousness it deserved, avoiding panic while embracing all the steps we could reasonably take to stay safe, following the data, and attempting to align our behavior with what our best information was telling us.

In short, our actions reflected the reality of the situation. Covid-19 was a disaster but not, fortunately, an apocalypse. Even as the mortality rate was unacceptably high, there was no sense that we faced global depopulation of the kind that remakes economic systems and shakes the foundations of core religious and political institutions. As a result, we chose to treat the disease like a significant threat, but not like a comet hurtling toward earth or a tsunami crashing into our shores. There were times when it could be said that elements of our response were characterized by overreaction, but it must also be said that we tried not to slide off the road of rationality and common sense, and our choices reflected this.

The common link between these choices—how we chose to think of the virus and how we chose to respond to it—is that we made them in a context of incomplete information. Here is a partial list of all we did not know at the start of the pandemic: initially, we knew very little about how the disease manifests and spreads; we did not know the extent to which its spread would be shaped by existing health inequities; and we did not—could not—know the long-term effects of the Covid-19 lockdown or of the virus itself. Nevertheless, we did not let our lack of perfect knowledge stop us from acting as quickly and decisively as we could when faced with Covid-19. Because here is what we did know: we knew that regardless of the scenario this novel pathogen presented, failure on our part to act could have meant we were hit with the worst case of it; we knew we needed to flatten the epidemic curve in order to maintain the capacity of health systems; we knew that, in addition to the physical health costs of the pandemic, there would also be mental health consequences; and while we did not know exactly how existing health inequities would shape the spread of Covid-19, we knew that they would play a role in helping contagion take hold in society, because they always do.

So at the start of Covid-19 we found ourselves in a gray area between knowledge and ignorance. Operating in this area, making decisions with incomplete data, was a necessary response to an unprecedented crisis. But it is also, in many ways, a common practice in science and public health. Figure 11.1 is an adaptation of the Knowledge to Action (K2A) Framework for Public Health, produced by the CDC's National Center for Chronic Disease Prevention and Health Promotion. It reflects the ideal process by which research might be tested, its results classified as useful knowledge, and this knowledge disseminated and, ultimately, institutionalized to inform the decisions that shape health. A key feature of this process is its length. First come the many steps that characterize the research phase; then, if the research is promising, a choice is made to translate that knowledge into practice. If its practical application is successful, the door opens for it to become institutionalized, where it may be regarded as a true best practice, of the type an organization such as the CDC or WHO might recommend for addressing challenges such as a pandemic.

It is important to stress, again, that this process represents the ideal. It is slow, painstaking, and deliberate. It arrives at its end through much trial and error, debate, and practical application. It is from this slow process that facts emerge—in marked contrast to the often-instantaneous process that generates opinions. It is easy to see how we might always want to make decisions that are supported by such a clearly defined process. This is even more understandable when lives hang in the balance. But the very length of this process means we cannot always apply these steps to every choice we make. A feature of crises is that they tend to appear suddenly. Sometimes we can apply part of this process—incorporating, for example, emerging but untested science

KNOWLEDGE TO ACTION FRAMEWORK FOR PUBLIC HEALTH

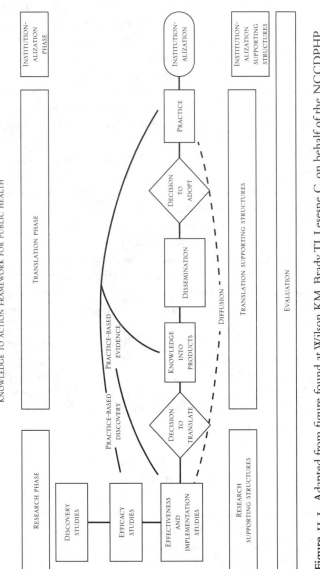

Figure 11.1.1. Adapted from figure found at Wilson KM, Brady TJ, Lesesne C, on behalf of the NCCDPHP Work Group on Translation. An Organizing Framework for Translation in Public Health: The Knowledge to Action Framework. *Preventing Chronic Disease.* 2011; 8(2): A46. Public domain.

into our view of the situation—but rarely can we apply all of its steps to the complex and fast-evolving circumstances of an acute challenge.

The experience of Covid-19 was marked by such complexity. The virus was just the beginning. The social, economic, and political effects of the contagion would have been daunting even without the added factor of a presidential election and, later, a national reckoning with the challenge of racial injustice. Then there was the new media environment, the polarization of opinion and the widespread skepticism of scientific authorities that had been so heightened during the Trump era, and the general feeling of acceleration that characterized world events in the latter half of the 2010s. This complexity meant that just when we began to feel we could apply a measure of certainty to something, circumstances would shift and we would have to reconsider all we thought we knew.

Such complexity can give rise to a sense of ambiguity, which can be disorienting if we are not used to it. We are, of course, constantly encountering ambiguity throughout our lives, yet the condition of the present moment—in particular, the emergence of new technologies—has amplified the complexity that makes it difficult to know where we stand in relation to our changing world. Take, for example, one of the more complex influences on our society today: the role of social media in our lives. There was a time when it was possible to believe we had a clear understanding of social media's effects. That time was roughly 2015. In 2015, social media had existed in its present form for about a decade, enough time for us to feel we had a sense of how it was shaping culture and the public conversation. The standard read on social media was that it was, broadly speaking, a positive influence. Certainly, there were concerns about privacy and data security, but on balance it seemed as though social media had democratized the public debate and helped to better connect the world. Politically, its central influence seemed to be its capacity to facilitate the rise of pro-democracy movements such as the Arab Spring.

Five years later, in 2020, the picture was more complex. The 2016 election revealed how social media can help spread misinformation and reinforce partisan echo chambers. Social media also did much to amplify conspiracy theories and skepticism of science and expertise in general, so when Covid-19 emerged, it did so in a context where millions of people were disinclined to believe anything that came from the mouths of so-called elites. This is not to say social media was revealed as a wholly negative force. Much of its potential as a democratizing, liberating influence remains, serving as a necessary counter to its less positive aspects. What this means, then, is that social media, with its dynamism and complexity, is an ambiguous influence, one that is constantly changing and resists definitive categorization. It has been fascinating to see how, in a polarized era where a common pastime has been to divide the world into categories of what we love and what we hate, social media has remained one of the few influences about which we still do not know quite what to think, where even those who decry the evils of Big Tech do so from their Twitter or Facebook account.

The complexities of social media reflect the complexities of the era into which Covid-19 emerged. It was a dynamic time, both democratic and tribalized, driven by technology, with the abundance of information provided by the internet and captured by smartphones leaving us not much closer to truth, and in some cases further away than we were in even the recent past. We were—and, in many ways, still are—finding our feet in this era. The virus added a new layer to the complexity of this moment. Navigating the pandemic meant navigating this complexity. It meant finding ourselves in a place of doubt, uncertainty, and change and working out a way to move forward.

Places of doubt, uncertainty, and change are not the most comfortable of places to be. Human beings tend to desire certainty. Indeed, we seem hardwired for it. We divide the world into clear distinctions, categorizing what we encounter as right or wrong, hazardous or helpful, organized or chaotic, intelligent or foolish, a pleasure or a pain. We likely do this in part because once we have categorized something, we then have an established means of engaging with it. We may not know much about something on first encounter, but we do know we have a mental framework for reacting to something that is good or something that is bad, something that helps or something that hinders. It is not necessary, then, to fully understand something—all we need to do is decide which familiar box to put it in, then regard it as we regard everything else in the box. We have become so used to doing this that we are even liable to mistake this shortcut, this process of categorization, for true knowledge of a subject.

This is perhaps an unflattering sketch of how our minds often function, but is it untrue? The Covid-19 era provided many examples of this tendency at work. The pandemic happened to coincide with a robust public debate about the issue of "cancel culture," in which opprobrium is directed against people whose statements or beliefs do not coincide with those of a particular political in-group. Often the effort to cancel someone stemmed from a belief that the target of this opprobrium was, through her words and thoughts, posing a threat to a marginalized or vulnerable population. As the debate over cancel culture unfolded, it engaged with the question of whether these targets were perpetrating actual harms or merely expressing political or cultural heterodoxies. The conversation about cancel culture was informed by a number of high-profile journalists leaving their jobs at various news outlets as a consequence of the ideological distance between themselves and the prevailing political viewpoint at their former publication. These departures reflected the broader polarization of opinion over core issues at that time, as well as the "with us or against us" attitude characterizing debate across the political spectrum.

Raising the issue of cancel culture, polarization, and political group-think may seem like a departure from the issues we have been discussing, but I would argue they reflect something core to our collective relationship to ambiguity, doubt, and complexity. They suggest how uncomfortable many of us are with these fundamental elements of life, how quick we are to attempt to expel or escape them. Rather than engage with complexity, ambiguity, and a sense of doubt informed by the possibility that our views might be wrong, we seek to put ideas and those espousing them into familiar categories of villainy or virtue. We try to distance ourselves from ambiguity—either by casting out those with whom we disagree or creating spaces where we can be sure we will not encounter them. Working to change this approach to ambiguity is working against what often seems like our core nature—the way we simplify the world in order to make sense of it. This is a challenging but necessary task if we are to cultivate the perspective that helps us build a healthier world.

We can find assistance in this work by listening to a perhaps unexpected voice: that of the poet John Keats. In a letter to his brothers, Keats expressed what he considered a key quality of "a man of achievement." He referred to this quality as "negative capability," and characterized it as "when man is capable of being in uncertainties, Mysteries, doubts, without any irritable reaching after fact & reason." Keats had trained as a surgeon and would have been familiar with the scientific process and the knowledge it produces. Yet in expressing what he saw as the most desirable cast of mind, he described the capacity to be comfortable amid "uncertainties, mysteries, doubts." This is not to say one should not aspire to gain the knowledge that can reduce uncertainty, only that we should be able to be at ease when circumstances are ambiguous, to retain the equanimity that allows us to make good decisions even when the way forward is unclear.

The marginalization of voices with which we might not agree, or the rush to place them in familiar categories, suggests how difficult achieving this ease can be. It also raises the issue of bias, one of the key impediments to the clear understanding that helps us navigate complexity. Biases can be easy to overlook, yet it is the rare individual who does not have them. They skew how we see the world, subtly shading our perceptions. Their influence is not always negative, of course. What is love, for example, if not a strong bias in favor of those about whom we care? Likewise, it would be difficult to advance any form of progress in the world without bias toward certain social, economic, and political systems. But bias becomes problematic when it prevents us from seeing a situation accurately. When this occurs, it becomes all the more difficult to pursue solutions that align with reality. During Covid-19, our biases made it harder for us to engage with a clear picture of the situation, informing our response in ways that at times were counterproductive.

We have already touched on some of the social and political inflections of such biases and their effect on our behavior during Covid-19. It is also worth mentioning how biases unfolded in the media, influencing public perception of events. An analysis of the tone of Covid-19-related English-language news articles found the tone of 91 percent of pieces by major media outlets in the United States was negative, whereas in non-US major sources coverage was 54 percent negative. In scientific journals, for their part, the tone was 65 percent negative. Notably, US media negativity persisted even in the context of positive developments such as vaccine trials, and remained unaffected by changing trends in case rates. This bias toward negativity was captured, for example, by the fact that there were more stories among major US media outlets about President Trump's dubious touting of the therapeutic powers of hydroxychloroquine than about companies and individual researchers working to develop Covid-19 vaccines.

Now, make no mistake: Covid-19 was a disaster and so warranted negative coverage. However, when this negativity was unrelenting, even in the face of good news, it created impressions that were not always accurate, which could have caused missteps in our approach to the virus. We have already discussed, for example, how embracing complete and perpetual lockdowns created a socioeconomic context that threatened health just as much as the virus did. It is difficult to think media bias against a more nuanced view of Covid-19 did not play a role in resisting a balanced approach to the lockdown.

The problem of bias reflects the broader challenge of facing ambiguity. Our biases emerge, in part, from our wish to find certainties in an uncertain world. When faced with ambiguity, it is human nature to try to find something about it to which we can attach certainty; failing that, we are inclined to turn away. Except that sometimes we cannot turn away. Life is full of times when we are forced to make choices based on incomplete knowledge. When weighing two job opportunities, for example, it is not always clear which would be the best one to take. As much as we might research a company, we cannot know everything about what it would be like to work there without actually working there, so in the end we must choose based on the knowledge we have. Or consider the decision of whether or not to have children. It is impossible to fully weigh all the variables at play in such a choice. While we may think we can imagine the economic, emotional, and physical demands of having kids—and the equally complex and surprising ways in which these demands are balanced by joy and love—anyone who has chosen to have children will likely admit it would not have been possible to fully appreciate these factors in advance of making this decision. All we can do in such situations is use what we do know to make the best possible choices. There is no escaping these decisions; even the decision not to choose is itself a choice.

When Covid-19 emerged, we did not have the option of not choosing—of doing nothing just because we did not know enough. Choosing not to act decisively to address the contagion could have meant facing a version of the pandemic that was even worse than what we experienced. Figure 11.2 is a visualization of potential epidemic curves, with and without protective measures. It is from a news article published early in the pandemic. While we did not know nearly as much then as we would later, it is clear we did know that failure to embrace protective measures would likely place the curve well above healthcare system capacity, with dire consequences. So we chose to act accordingly.

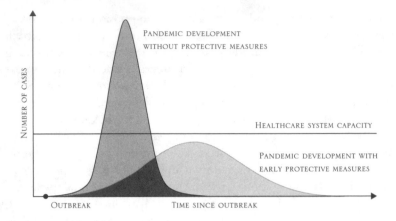

Figure 11.2. Adapted from figure found at Roberts S. Flattening the Coronavirus Curve. *The New York Times*. March 27, 2020. https://www.nytimes.com/article/flatten-curve-coronavirus.html. Accessed January 4, 2021.

Regardless of what form the virus would ultimately take, whether it was another Black Death or merely a slightly worse version of the flu, we knew in the moment of its emergence that we needed to make some major changes to how our society operates in order to keep the epidemic curve as flat as possible. It was also clear that these changes would involve sacrifice. Figure 11.3 visualizes the spike in unemployment claims in the United States during March 2020. It is a snapshot of the immediate economic costs of the pandemic, with 3.3 million Americans filing for unemployment in just one week.

As we have discussed, such economic costs are not incidental to public health; they are, in fact, integral to it. Economic shocks like what we experienced during Covid-19 generate sickness and death just as surely as a hurricane striking a city or a virus spreading like wildfire does. In accepting the short-term economic costs of a lockdown, we were accepting what we hoped would be the lesser of two evils. We took steps we knew would result in sickness and death in order to prevent a potentially worse catastrophe. In this sense, it was not unlike decisions made during wartime. In a war, leaders will often make decisions about troop deployments and battle plans that they know will result in the deaths of their own soldiers. Sometimes they

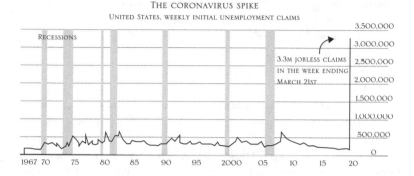

Figure 11.3. Adapted from figure found at The Coronavirus Has Pushed 3.3m American Workers onto the Dole in a Week. *The Economist*. March 26, 2020. https://www.economist.com/graphic-detail/2020/03/26/the-coronavirus-has-pushed-33m-american-workers-onto-the-dole-in-a-week. Accessed January 4, 2021.

know these numbers will be tragically high. During the Civil War, for example, Ulysses S. Grant, when in command of Union forces, would make choices that he knew would result in the death of thousands of his own men. During World War II, Dwight Eisenhower, in command on the eve of D-Day, knew that the Allied invasion of German-occupied Western Europe would come at a terrible cost. But these commanders pressed forward anyway, because they believed the plans they chose would prevent a far worse outcome—the triumph of an evil cause. It may seem inappropriate to compare these choices to decisions that affect the conditions that shape health, but I would argue that the comparison is entirely apt, and the fact that this is not apparent to all reflects how far we still have to go in our approach to health. Covid-19 killed more Americans, by far, than the Vietnam War. The sickness and death caused by the economic consequences of this moment will likely be comparable to that of any number of wars and large-scale military engagements. Decisions about health directly shape the pattern of such mortality. The late William Bicknell, a professor of global health at Boston University and something of a legend in the field, used to define public health as "the art and science of deciding who dies, when, and with what degree of misery." There is a battlefield quality to this statement, which is apt. Promoting health is about making trade-offs. The long-term goal of public health is to create a world where no one sickens or dies a preventable death. In the short term, however, decisions about health are often less about ensuring no one dies and more about creating a context where the fewest possible die. This involves making choices like the ones we made at the start of Covid-19.

Another way in which such choices reflect those made during war is the context in which they are considered. The conditions of confusion, doubt, and incomplete knowledge are the natural habitat of military decision-makers. These conditions are what is meant by the phrase "the fog of war." Military choices are regularly made by leaders with limited knowledge of their enemy's capabilities and plans, the state of the terrain, and many other factors that could prove decisive when the battle is joined. In order to be effective, the people making these choices must be comfortable working in complexity, ambiguity, and doubt. They must thrive on it. It is in the nature of their work to analyze the information at their disposal, acknowledge where it is incomplete, and act decisively, with the understanding that their choices may often reflect "the least-worst option." In doing so, they must strike a balance. They must not tip over into arrogance, thinking they know more than they do, courting the fall the comes with such pride. Nor can they be so overwhelmed by the many factors at play that they risk timidity, panicked overreaction, or outright dereliction of duty.

These were the same risks we faced at the start of Covid-19 and which we face in every decision that affects the health of populations. In making these choices, we also face roughly the same trade-offs as those inherent in a plan for military action. There was no way to implement a mass lockdown without causing widespread economic harm, and there was no way to cause widespread economic harm without hurting people. We knew this, but we also knew that failure to act could hurt far more. These core facts, these areas where our knowledge was secure, were enough to outweigh the many other unknowns and show us the way forward.

Our choice to embrace a lockdown can seem like a unique event, emerging from an unprecedented crisis. The trade-off we made, accepting economic pain in exchange for preventing a Covid-19 nightmare scenario, can appear in hindsight almost as historically singular as the pandemic itself. Yet the truth is that we make such choices, with their attendant trade-offs, all the time. Whenever we make choices about the large-scale forces that shape health, we are—when the choice is stripped to its essence—making a choice about who lives and who dies. When such choices undermine health, their effects can be deep and widespread. This can be the result of policymakers choosing to deprioritize health or of corporations placing profits before the well-being of communities, or it need not be anything so deliberate. As seen with the wreck of the *Méduse*, the choice to accept political dysfunction and socioeconomic drift can be just as damaging as any targeted harm.

Given the constant necessity of making choices that shape health on a large scale, it is important that we become comfortable with the conditions of complexity and doubt that often characterize this decision-making process. At the same time, we need a science that supports an understanding of what matters most for health, so that we can minimize the number of unknowns and be as clear as possible about the trade-offs inherent in the choices we make. Aspiring to be comfortable with complexity and doubt does not mean we should embrace ignorance or give up on ever knowing anything fully. Instead, we need to embrace Keats's "negative capability" as a supplement to the ongoing work of trying to deepen our understanding of the forces that shape health.

During Covid-19, this meant acting on what we knew while adapting to the situation as it evolved. As we have discussed, in the pandemic's latter months, when we knew more about the disease, there was a balance to be struck between shutting down much of society while also keeping open certain critical sectors where the data did not reflect significant Covid-19 spread. This balance was not available to us in the early days of the pandemic. We needed to give healthcare providers the space to do their work, and we needed to buy time in order to better understand the disease so we could emerge from the lockdown with new data-informed tools for addressing it. Faced with the complexity of an evolving situation and our own incomplete knowledge, we made our choice, and accepted the trade-offs it would entail. As we learned more about the virus, however, it became necessary for us to update our approach, to bring it in line with new information. Working in complexity means engaging with the fluidity of a situation as new information becomes known. This was where we floundered during Covid-19. We were slow to adapt to what the data were telling us about the disease and remained entrenched in our ideological camps, with some digging in their heels on perpetual lockdowns and others refusing to give an inch on acting as if the pandemic did not exist. This prevented us from being as nimble as we should have been, hindering our ability to respond to the pandemic. So we were left with an uneven situation where certain regions—such as the Cherokee Nation—did well during Covid-19 while others did poorly, rather than a uniformly effective response guided by an ability to adapt in the face of complexity and change.

Our uneven response to the pandemic reflects a core truth about engaging with complexity: it is difficult to do. It is important to acknowledge this. Engaging with complexity is hard, and while this does not absolve us when we stumble, it is a fact that must be considered in our post-Covid-19 self-evaluation. Complexity can be so difficult to engage with that there is an entire field dedicated to becoming better at doing so. This field is known as systems science. Systems science is the study of the complex networks found in nature, in economies, in communities, in science and technology, and in the forces that give rise to health. I have spent much of my career exploring how systems science can improve our understanding of these forces. To study systems science is to be constantly reminded of how outcomes such as health are rarely, if ever, a product of single causes. They are, in fact, deeply shaped by an interplay of forces—a dynamic, constantly evolving network of complexity that we must learn to navigate, toward the aim of improving health.

This requires us to continually ask the question posed in Chapter 10: what matters most? In parsing complexity, we need to be able to discern which factors matter most to health, and act decisively to engage with them. This reflects the importance of values in our approach to health. Values can help us navigate complexity and doubt in the face of incomplete information, shaping an approach to health rooted in what matters most. Complexity can seem, at times, like part of the storm that tosses our ship, threatening to throw us off course. To navigate this, we must turn to the values that function as the stars that help us orient ourselves in whatever situation we face. When we embrace a set of core values around health, we have a means of charting our course regardless of the weather. The difficulty is arriving at a set of values we can all share. We all agree we want to be healthy, but we do not all agree on the values that animate a healthy society. We saw this during the pandemic, as it became clear that for some, health meant just the absence of disease, while for others, it meant access to the full range of socioeconomic resources that enable health. Choosing between these two approaches is an example of just the type of decision that brings us into contact with complexity and doubt.

We should choose an approach to health that is based on the pursuit of the conditions we have been discussing in this book: the conditions that make health possible. For example, during Covid-19 we often heard that we faced a choice between the economy, on one hand, and health, on the other. But a society that values health enough to truly understand it would know this is a false choice. Economics is just as deeply tied to health as the advance of disease is. In the long term, in fact, economics can be even more significant for health. When we understand this, we can make better decisions. The same is true when we understand the full range of conditions that shape health—from the design of cities to the governmental policies that affect the food we eat, the water we drink, and the air we breathe. When we value these conditions as a means of supporting health, we have a basis for sound decision-making when crisis strikes.

Our values, then, are what can guide us when our knowledge is incomplete, our circumstances ambiguous. When we decide that we value health, and we understand that valuing health means not just avoiding disease but supporting the foundational structures that generate well-being, we have a template for action in the face of complexity. It is worth noting here that values are not the same as ideology. If values are like stars for us to follow—allowing for maneuvering and improvising in a changing context of challenge and uncertainty—ideology can lead to inflexibility and even abuses in pursuit of an ideal. We encountered this during Covid-19, as ideological rigidity prevented us from taking all of the steps necessary for safeguarding health. Too often, we saw the phenomenon of people deciding well in advance how they would choose to think about the pandemic, a choice more often informed by preexisting ideological narratives than by the evolving reality of the data or concern for the core forces that shape health. For these people, a change of opinion about the best steps to take necessitated not merely changing one's mind to align with the data but changing an entire worldview—a much different, and more difficult, proposition. Facing complexity, then, we are best served by values that can inform our actions, rather than by ideologies that dictate them. It is important, always, to stay open-minded and nimble when dealing with ambiguity and doubt, guided by values that prioritize creating stronger foundations for health.

How can we promote an understanding that embraces, as core values, improving the conditions that support health? One of the key steps we can take is engaging with the public conversation to spread awareness of the true foundations of health; I will talk about this more in Chapter 12. Even more fundamentally, we can get to these values by following what the science says about the conditions that shape health. Throughout this book, we have looked at data that reflect the deep and complex links between health and the fabric of our world. While these links are not always clear to the general public, they are inescapable in even a cursory review of the scientific literature about health. During Covid-19, the researchers and public health experts who regularly engage with this science were at the center of the national conversation, with many becoming household names. Their words, their guidance, helped us navigate the complexity of the moment. We should not stop listening to them now that Covid-19 has passed. Nor should we allow ourselves to lose interest in the science we once followed on a near-hourly basis back when doing so could mean the difference between life and death, sickness and health. We need to keep this science at the heart of our national conversation, so that it can inform our culture and our values and we can shift toward the deeper understanding of health that can support a better future. While the complexities of dealing with Covid-19 may have passed, complexity remains at the heart of the forces that shape health. Becoming comfortable with complexity will only become more important as we set aside our simplistic, healthcare-centric view of health and engage with these broader forces.

12

Humility and Informing
the Public Conversation

I will end this book on what may seem like a strange note—by discussing the importance of humility in preventing the contagion next time. Humility is not something we often think about when envisioning how we can shape a better world. Changing the world is a pursuit we tend to associate with thinking big, with the boundless ambition we regard as necessary for accomplishing major progress. Yet humility is, in fact, core to the success of these efforts. At the same time, shaping a healthier world means informing a public conversation that prioritizes what matters most for health. It means elevating the subjects we have been discussing in this book to the center of our national conversation about health, a conversation currently focused on the curative power of medicine at the expense of the forces that shape health. In this task, too, humility is key. Humility helps us to listen and engage with respect, compassion, and an openness to alternative perspectives. Throughout Covid-19, we saw how hubris and closed-minded partisanship undermined, again and again, the possibility of such a conversation, hindering our efforts to support health. Going forward, we need an approach to health that embraces humility and constructive engagement with the public conversation, toward the aim of building a healthier world.

Looking back at how this conversation unfolded during Covid-19, we are faced with many examples of how the pandemic might have had a humbling effect on our thinking. One of the key features of Covid-19 was that during the pandemic almost everyone was wrong about something. Some were wrong about how long the pandemic would last. Others were wrong about the deadliness of the disease. Still

others were wrong about how long it would take to produce a vaccine, or about the protective virtues of masks. I, personally, was wrong
about the extent to which scientific recommendations would become
politicized during the crisis. Some politicization was to be expected,
of course, but I was truly surprised to see something as basic as mask-
wearing during a pandemic become a partisan flashpoint.

One of the reasons so many were wrong about so much is our
tendency, discussed in Chapter 11, to seek certainty in the face of complex, ambiguous situations. In the face of an unprecedented threat,
with a range of possible outcomes, there is comfort in being able to
say about certain possible outcomes, "This much we can predict," even
when the broader trajectory of a situation remains anyone's guess. In
offering predictions, however, we make ourselves hostages to fortune,
and fortune often twists and turns in ways that prove us wrong. This
was the case for many of us during Covid-19.

This is not to say, of course, that we should not have done our
best to envision how the crisis would unfold. It is necessary to make
informed predictions as we navigate challenge. It is worth noting, too,
that not all of the predictions we made during Covid-19 were off-base.
There was, for example, the relative confidence many had throughout
the pandemic that a vaccine would eventually be developed, even as
the speed with which this was accomplished was a welcome surprise.
Then there was the widely shared early understanding that whatever
the novel coronavirus was, it was not the flu and should not be treated
as such. Yet, despite our successful projections, few of us can look back
on the year of the pandemic as a time of complete, surefooted success
in everything we said and did.

These missteps reflected our limitations in understanding and influencing the world and the conditions that shape it. They were remind-
ers that, for all our knowledge, what we do not know will likely always
outweigh what we do. The virus, too, was a reminder of this. It was
far bigger than any of us, and its presence in our lives highlighted
socioeconomic conditions that are bigger still. Facing these forces, we
could do little as individuals—it was only through our collective effort,
imperfect as it was, that we were able to muddle through the crisis.
The very imperfections of this effort reinforced the lesson of limits,
as did the ultimate reminder of our finite capacities: death. The presence of death—always there but, in our society, only intermittently
acknowledged—was the central feature of the pandemic. It was what

we feared, what we went to such great lengths to avoid, what lay at the heart of all we did during those troubled months. Because so much of the Covid-19 mortality was concentrated among certain vulnerable populations, it was possible to make it through the pandemic without a sense of the sheer scope of the death. Emergency room physician Cleavon Gilman, formerly a combat medic deployed with the Marines in Iraq, said of the pandemic, "I've trained for this. I've been in war, and this is absolutely worse. There are no borders in this war. There is no date when I know I'm going home." A December 2020 *STAT News* piece about his experience treating patients during the pandemic reflected how unprecedented the mortality caused by Covid-19 truly was. "Seeing this kind of death is not normal," Gilman said.

Proximity to death and the realization of our own mistakes were perhaps the key enforcers during the pandemic of the importance of humility. I say "enforcers" because humility is not something toward which we are always naturally inclined to turn. It is far easier to turn toward pride, toward achievement, toward our sense of unlimited human potential. Turning toward humility can, on the other hand, be difficult, and it often takes a personal or collective blow to shake us out of our easy triumphalism. Covid-19 was such a blow. It forced us to confront how we are subject to influences larger than ourselves, influences over which we have little control as individuals, influences that deeply shape our health.

But humility is more than something that tempers our pride. It is an essential tool for building a healthier world, a world that is resistant to contagion. Humility helps us to lay the foundation of knowledge necessary for putting in place structures that generate health. It seems perhaps paradoxical to suggest that we cannot advance knowledge without a keen sense of the limits of what we know. Yet this is precisely the case. One of the core principles of the scientific pursuit of knowledge is epistemic humility—the notion that our inquiries should be informed by the understanding that "we do not know what we do not know." To embrace epistemic humility is to bear in mind the words derived from Plato's telling of the life of Socrates: "I know that I know nothing." This speaks to the idea that a healthy awareness of our own ignorance is fundamental to our pursuit of knowledge. After all, if we think we know everything, what reason do we have to learn more? If we are convinced our worldview is accurate in every respect, why should we leave our minds open to new perspectives and ideas?

The humility that comes with a sense of the limits of our knowledge is particularly important in an era when the politicization of key issues threatens, at times, the possibility of open, honest conversation. I touched on this in Chapter 11 in addressing the issue of cancel culture and the polarization of the public debate. A conversation that is hostile to complexity and informed by rigid ideological certainties is not one that can inform a healthier world. This is not to say, of course, that engaging in the public conversation from a place of humility means compromising core values, only that we must always be open to the possibility that we might be wrong, and that the person with whom we are engaging may be able to shed light on some key points that we ourselves have missed.

This is also not to say we should disregard everything we think we know or give up on the idea of objective truths we can consistently apply to solving real-world problems. That would be absurd. Certainly, core scientific principles—the principles of flight, for example—need no second-guessing. We know they work. But the broader paradigms in which they operate, the worldviews that inform their application— these are worth constant reappraisal. We know the principles of flight work, but what about our ideas about how these principles are applied? For decades, for example, we have been fairly complacent about applying them to the future of space travel. We have embraced a paradigm in which space exploration has been the province of governments, with the assumption that they were the entities best capable of funding and coordinating such a massive undertaking. In recent years, however, some people, notably Elon Musk (to return to him, giving him his due after earlier criticism), have questioned these assumptions and argued for a robust program of commercial spaceflight in which reusable spacecraft could someday, and perhaps sooner than we think, make us a multiplanetary species. Such ambition may seem a product of hubris, but on closer examination it is possible to see how it may be informed by a radical humility, which creates space for the possibility that we do not know nearly enough about space travel—or, indeed, about our own technological potential—to make assumptions about what is and is not possible in this area. Likewise, while what I am calling for in this book—the reorganization of society in the interest of health—may seem overly ambitious, it emerges from a willingness to accept that we do not fully grasp our own capacity to evolve in the face of necessity, to meet the challenges we face. It is both a paradox and the truth that, sometimes, pursuing the boldest ambition is possible only in a context of deep humility.

This is perhaps best understood when considering the realm of art. It is often the case that the most successful artists, the ones who remain creative and relevant over a long career, are those who are most humble about their craft. This is not to say they might not have egos, only that, when it comes to the work they produce, they are driven by a recognition that art is bigger than any one artist. The artists at the very top of their profession are the ones who are humble enough to let the work take possession of them rather than approach the fundamental creative force as something they can somehow master on their own. They are skilled enough to see just how vast the forces they are dealing with really are, and it is the sense of engaging with these larger forces that keeps them going, keeps them surprising.

This was apparent in some of the creative output we saw in the year of Covid-19. During the pandemic, Bob Dylan, then in his late seventies, released a new album. It received excellent reviews and generated much enthusiasm, with many hailing it as having brought some light and perspective to a dark time. The public seemed grateful to be hearing from this most American of voices at a moment when the United States was facing one of its greatest challenges. Just as Dylan's songs characterized the turbulent 1960s when he first emerged as an artist, his new album, *Rough and Rowdy Ways*, was praised for reflecting the essence of our society in a troubled age. Reviewers remarked how impressive it was that Dylan was still releasing work at such a high level at a time in life when many consider retiring. Core to his ability to do so, arguably, is his capacity to remain humble in relation to his art, despite his many achievements. He displayed this humility when he received the 2016 Nobel Prize in Literature. Recipients of the prize are required to give a public lecture, and Dylan's was about the tradition from which his work emerged. He spoke with an implicit humility of the songs, books, and poems that influenced him, focusing less on his life story as an entertainer and more on the age-old sources of his art. It was clear in the speech that he saw himself not as a master of this tradition but as its conduit, as a vessel for larger forces. This was evident in his choice to close the lecture with a version of a line from Homer, "Sing in me, oh Muse, and through me tell the story."

We, too, are dealing with larger forces—the forces that shape health. For our engagement with these forces to be most effective, it must proceed from a place of humility. If we do not proceed with humility, we risk pursuing the wrong priorities, doubling down on our scientific work around medicine and neglecting the conditions that shape health. Because it is in the realm of science where we are perhaps least likely to have humility—and for not unjustifiable reasons. The end of Covid-19 was in many ways a scientific triumph, the speed with which we found a vaccine—indeed, multiple vaccines—suggesting the limitless potential of biomedical research. Our triumphalism about this work is valid, and the potential of this area of research for generating further advances is undeniable. It is easy to feel that if we can accomplish feats like the speedy development of the Covid-19 vaccine, the time when we achieve something resembling complete scientific knowledge cannot be far off. When this time comes, in theory we can use this knowledge to end disease for good. To return to the parallel with space exploration, the world just after the development of a Covid-19 vaccine perhaps felt a bit like how the world felt after the first moon landing—dazzled by the possibilities of the technology that brought about this achievement. After the moon landing, it would have been easy to think, "If we could do this less than a hundred years after the development of the airplane, surely the day cannot be far off when we can use this technology to travel to distant worlds." After the swift development of a Covid-19 vaccine, we may well feel something similar—as though the end of all disease might actually be possible through advances in drugs and treatments.

Yet such aspirations do not necessarily lead to desired outcomes. As of this writing, we have not achieved the dream of sending humans to other planets. Likewise, the triumph of vaccines does not mean the inevitable end of disease. The truth is that treatment can carry us only so far. To build the healthier world that will truly prevent the emergence of disease, we must engage with the forces that shape health, in all their complexity. This starts with being humble in our approach to these forces, recognizing that while we can influence them through our collective effort and investment, they are not some mountain we can climb, nor a moon on which we can plant a flag. We cannot "master," in any meaningful way, the forces that shape health. We can only engage with them, guided by the best possible data, with the aim of channeling their influence into better health. It is like irrigation, by which farmers redirect water flows to nourish crops. In doing so, they are not conquering the great rivers whose water they draw. Rather, they are using their technological know-how to work in cooperation with them, bearing in mind that at any moment the river could flood, a dam could break, or something else could happen to turn the waters from a helpful resource into a destructive force. This awareness helps the farmer remain humble in her engagement with the waters that have such power to shape her life. The same awareness should characterize our approach to the forces that influence health.

A key impediment to this humility is what we discussed in Chapter 11: our aversion to ambiguity and complexity. These factors, and the feeling of doubt they often inform, are a hallmark of dealing with the larger forces that shape health. If we let them, they help us maintain a sense of proportion relative to these forces, and are the companions of any honest effort to reckon with the foundations of health. Our discomfort with complexity and ambiguity, and our consequent preference for the seemingly simpler option of ending disease through medicine alone, reflects why we need humility, why it is a prerequisite for the work we must do to build a healthier world.

One of the reasons we are so uncomfortable with the experience of complexity and ambiguity is that we tend to see it as a temporary state, a detour on the road to the complete knowledge we feel our scientific understanding will ultimately deliver. Believing this, we see no reason to get comfortable with the feeling of doubt and incomplete knowledge, because why get used to something we believe to be temporary? Yet this belief has not served us well, as Covid-19 amply illustrated. We should not allow the development of vaccines to cause us to forget that while the story of the pandemic ended with the triumph of medical science, the tale, in its entirety, was overwhelmingly one of the failures of our current, medicine-obsessed approach to health. The reason the race for a vaccine needed to be a race at all was because we allowed our society to become a place where contagion could easily take hold. We did this in large part by lavishing money and focus on creating better drugs and treatments while neglecting the socioeconomic conditions that shape health. Our pursuit of these treatments is, I would argue, a proxy for our pursuit of certainty. When we think of a drug, we are thinking of something we see as dependable, simple. We are thinking of what is essentially a button we can push when we are sick that we can be reasonably sure will quickly make us well. Notably, drugs fulfill the function of cure without any of the messy encounters with our own societal shortcomings involved in the process of building a healthier world. It is not hard to see how this might be appealing—it is the certainty of cure without the ambiguities inherent in prevention. Yet through our pursuit of total certainty and our confidence that we can one day attain it, we have put off creating a world that is less vulnerable to poor health. We have advanced a fantasy of perfect cure, and made the perfect the enemy of the good, of the progress necessary for building a healthier world. To advance this progress, we need humility.

The importance of humility is clear when we take a closer look at just what our medical triumphalism was able to achieve during the pandemic. We should never forget that the world that gave us vaccines in record time also gave us, in the United States alone, hundreds of thousands of deaths and millions of Covid-19 cases. What was medicine able to do in the face of this? The honest answer is: relatively little. This is not to say it did nothing—far from it. The courage and skill of health workers and the rapid advance of better therapeutics were key to safeguarding the population during Covid-19, to reducing the mortality rate from what was an unknown disease in an incredibly brief period of time. This was all extraordinary. It would even be fair to call the time of the pandemic American medicine's finest hour. However, it is significant that even during this, its finest hour, medicine could not stop the pandemic from becoming a conflagration, overwhelming hospitals and funeral homes, touching every aspect of our lives. This is the fault not of medicine but of our willingness to prioritize medicine above all else in our approach to health. Not only does this approach undermine health but, as we have previously discussed, it even undermines medicine in the long run, by ensuring that the weight of our failure to adequately safeguard health will fall most heavily on our healthcare infrastructure when crisis strikes.

We have let this status quo persist because we thought we could, because we believed ourselves able to master disease rather than engage, with humility, with the forces that allow it to emerge. This miscalculation and its tragic consequences during Covid-19 reflect the darker side of the absence of humility—the rise of hubris. There is nothing wrong with pride in our medical abilities, a pride rooted in an honest appraisal of their strengths and limitations. But to turn toward hubris is to court the grandiose self-confidence that threatens to obscure an accurate assessment of what we can and cannot do. When this lack of vision meets the natural ambiguity of a crisis, the door is open for the kind of mistakes that cost many lives. We have now lived through such a crisis, and I do not just mean Covid-19. As I hope this book has shown, the long-standing conditions of our society, in which injustice and health inequities have allowed significant pockets of our population to face generations of preventable disease and death, constituted a crisis long before the spread of a novel pathogen beginning in 2019. Covid-19 was really a crisis on top of a crisis, exploiting the poor health that we, blinded by hubris, have allowed to proliferate in our society.

Think back, for example, to the life of Pamela Rush. Think about the poverty she endured, and how it was reflective of the poverty faced by millions of Americans in every state, even in the midst of our country's wealth. Think about the gap in life expectancy between white and Black Americans roughly 3.6 years. Imagine the level of hardship and injustice that goes into grinding 3.6 years off the life expectancy of a given group. It took the combined epidemics of suicide, drug overdose, and firearm violence to generate recent consecutive annual declines in overall US life expectancy, to say nothing of what Covid-19 will likely do to these numbers. The convergence of these challenges is relatively recent, lending historical uniqueness to the life expectancy declines we have seen. But the Black-white life expectancy gap is as old as the country itself, deeply persistent despite progress in narrowing it. It is a consequence of history and present-day socioeconomic inequity that we have long ignored, or at least insufficiently addressed. Can we really call this status quo anything other than a crisis?

The existence of such a crisis, in addition to being a problem to solve, is yet another reason for us to remain humble. Because as long as we accept injustice, no matter how advanced our technology or sky-high our aspirations, we will be marked as a country unwilling to correct the fundamental problems in our midst. That we should continue to be such a place should give us pause. For many people, the process of growing up involves sooner or later encountering some personal challenge or shortcoming that lays us low. This experience can temper our inclination toward pride and feelings of invulnerability informed by our capabilities, and open us to humility. An injury can do this, or an instance of being wrong about something deeply important. In the United States, we face a collective version of this in the health inequities we have allowed to persist—in particular, in the racial injustices that continue to undermine well-being in this country. Any honest appraisal of these shortcomings—which is, I hope, what is to be found in this book—should be cause for humility, a reminder that for all we can accomplish, we are also capable of the deepest failings. Given our potential for both the best and the worst, we should proceed humbly, improving what we can, correcting our mistakes, and not allowing a healthy appreciation of our potential to blind us to how we have failed to live up to it.

The challenges of vaccine distribution are a revealing snapshot of the crisis of health inequities within our society and how large this crisis looms, larger even than the accomplishment of the vaccines. As I have mentioned, distributing the vaccines meant having hard conversations about the vulnerability of certain populations compared to others, and about the socioeconomic conditions that shaped these vulnerabilities. A core debate in the early days of the vaccine was over whom to immunize first: the elderly or essential workers. On one hand, the elderly were by far the population most at risk of Covid-19. On the other hand, essential workers often come from the low-income communities of color that were disproportionately affected by the virus. The difficult conversation about these inequities, and the lack of simple solutions, is a reminder of the ambiguities inherent in dealing with the socioeconomic forces that shape health. It is also striking how, in addressing these deeper issues, the research and technologies that created the vaccines, and which represent so much of our thinking about health, are almost beside the point. Far more central to the conversation—indeed, far more central to the pandemic itself—are the underlying societal conditions that made the vaccine necessary in the first place.

In many ways, Covid-19 forced a reckoning with the realities of health. This reckoning raised the conditions that shape health to the level of prominence they deserve in the public debate, as seen in the conversation about vaccination. But there is still a tug-of-war happening, in which our hubris about the potential of treatment and our tendency to focus solely on the progress of science threaten to pull focus from these conditions and put it back where it has long been: on healthcare at the expense of health. This tug-of-war remains ongoing, and its outcome will determine whether or not we are as vulnerable to future events. Working to keep focus on what matters most for health will take patient engagement with the public debate. It will take a willingness to be honest about what happened during the pandemic and to learn the lessons of that moment. It will also take humility. We need to recognize the role that hubris played in leaving us vulnerable to the pandemic and realize the practical necessity of humility as a counterweight to our at times excessive pride.

Doing so has rarely been more important than it is now. Because while medical technology did little to prevent Covid-19 or temper its worst effects, its success in ending the pandemic was real, and, in some respects, unprecedented. Not only did it end the pandemic, but it allowed us to believe we did so entirely through our own scientific prowess. This created the conditions for our post-Covid-19 celebrations to be tinged by a sense of pride, potentially hubris, stemming from this achievement.

In late 2020, the journalist Andrew Sullivan wrote in an essay about the coming post-Covid-19 moment:

> The difference between this plague and every one before AIDS is that it didn't blow itself out. We put an end to it. The passivity and fatalism that marked many human experiences of plague are, in this moment, avoidable. We can rightly see this turning point as a real scientific breakthrough, with vast implications for tackling plague viruses in the future.

He wrote this as part of a piece celebrating the potential for a post-pandemic "Roaring Twenties," in which we begin the new decade on an optimistic note, buoyed by scientific success, a political and economic sea change, and an end to the isolation of lockdowns. Such a scenario would indeed be welcome. Yet it is also important to consider how this might contribute to the worst possible outcome in a post-pandemic world: forgetting about Covid-19. For individuals who lost friends and loved ones, of course, there can be no forgetting, no matter how celebratory a turn the culture takes in the wake of the virus. But for everyone else, there is a real danger that the upshot of this whole unprecedented experience will be putting it out of mind as quickly as possible. This collective forgetting may well be abetted by the vaccine, which, as Sullivan observed, allowed us to decisively end the crisis through our technical acumen. This decisiveness, welcome as it was, could have the double-edged effect of making it even easier for us to forget the lessons of the pandemic and leave in place the vulnerabilities that made Covid-19 so bad and could make future pandemics even worse.

Implicit in all this is the fact that while it seems, with Covid-19 behind us, like we have entered an era of safety, we have, in fact, entered a time of danger. In some ways, the post-pandemic era is even more perilous than the days of the virus, because our excitement at being "out of the woods" threatens to misdirect our focus, obscure the lessons of Covid-19, and leave us vulnerable to the even deadlier virus we know will come. We often see this in history, where a celebratory era following a moment of collective danger only serves as prologue to an even greater peril. This was the case during the original Roaring Twenties, when a time of cultural decadence and a desire to leave the grim war years behind informed the context from which World War II emerged. We also see this trope in literature, in which the celebrations that attend the end of one crisis mask the makings of the next calamity. This was the case, for example, in John Milton's epic poem *Paradise Lost*, which begins with the end of the war in heaven, in which Satan and his followers have been banished to hell after rebelling against God. In this sorry state, Satan schemes to take revenge for his defeat. The central disaster of the story—Satan's successful effort to cause Adam and Eve to eat fruit from the tree of the knowledge of good and evil—unfolds in this context as an action following a great conflict that was not as well resolved as it may have seemed.

We encounter similar plots in the work of Shakespeare, who was very interested in the pathologies that can take hold in communities in the immediate aftermath of wars. A number of his plays are set right after a great conflict has concluded, only to depict the rise of some terrible new threat that takes the characters by surprise. Examples of this include *Macbeth* and *Richard III*. The latter even starts with a speech where the protagonist expresses his alienation from the celebrations following the end of a civil war and his intention to use the complacency of the postwar days to set in motion a plot to seize the English crown for himself through subversion and murder. The speech begins with the famous lines "Now is the winter of our discontent / Made glorious summer by this sun of York."

It could well be said that now is the winter of *our* discontent made glorious summer by this "sun" of Moderna, Pfizer-BioNTech, Oxford-AstraZeneca, et cetera. This was even literally true when the vaccines were first introduced to the public, as the Covid-19 winter surge gave way to a summer of falling case rates and general relief. But there is another way our situation parallels Shakespeare. In *Richard III*, the playwright depicts Richard, Duke of Gloucester, who schemes for the crown. Born with physical deformities, he has become embittered due to a life of marginalization and abuse. At the start of the play, a series of dynastic conflicts, known as the Wars of the Roses, has elevated his brother Edward to power. The court is rejoicing at the end of the wars and the start of what everyone believes to be a new period of stability. What they have overlooked is Richard. All his life he has faced neglect and scorn, even amid the privilege of nobility. Right underneath the noses of his wealthy and powerful family, he has become an angry, conniving would-be tyrant, and he takes the end of the Wars of the Roses as his cue to commence a bloody quest for power, using the triumphalism of the moment to mask his designs until it is too late. Throughout the play, he kills men, women, and children everyone who stands between him and the crown—until he has finally accomplished his goal. In this, he is aided by the hubris and complacency of those around him, which prevent those who might have stopped him from fully seeing the danger they face.

We confront a similar danger now, in this post-Covid-19 moment. We have achieved a great victory over disease. But we should not confuse the end of one battle with the winning of a war. A vaccine has put the initial terror of Covid-19 behind us, but it has left in place the conditions that allow contagion to take hold. These conditions are roughly the same as those that created the threat of Richard, just on a larger scale. When, in a context of wealth and plenty, we allow certain communities to face marginalization and what amounts to socioeconomic abuse, when we overlook these communities for years, when we let this status quo persist even after an experience of shared danger that should have triggered our compassion for these groups, when all these missteps are enabled by a hubris that prevents us from seeing where we stumble, we have created the context for disaster to emerge. And just as the disaster of King Richard spared nobody, touching every demographic with the threat of a violent end, there is no guarantee the contagion next time will not strike with a lethality not seen since the era when Shakespeare himself was writing, when theaters were regularly closed due to the terror of plague.

This is what we could face if we allow ourselves to forget the lessons of Covid-19—if our scientific triumph informs a hubris that leads us to dismiss the conditions underlying health and instead double down on our investment in science-based cures. Such cures have long had the advantage of glamour, with their novelty and reliance on the latest, headline-friendly research. They now have the added advantage of being seen as the heroes of the Covid-19 moment. In explaining why this is problematic, it is important to stress that I do not mean to diminish the importance of medical science in general, nor its particular importance in ending Covid-19. Vaccines and those responsible for them were indeed among the heroes of the moment, and they deserve recognition. However, this recognition should not be allowed to distract from the necessary task of building a healthier world.

The reason it might indeed distract is that the steps needed to create such a world, the steps outlined in this book, are not, by and large, new or particularly glamorous. Taken together, they amount to a radical reimagining of our society. Individually, however, they are steps with which many of us are familiar. Better housing, a fairer economy, accessible quality education, a clean environment, the pursuit of social, economic, and racial justice—such measures have long been known to us as improvements that would better society. Perhaps their most novel characteristic, as presented in this book, is the idea of approaching them as part of a cohesive vision for health. But they are not as likely to attract the same level of hype-driven interest as cutting-edge biomedical research. Addressing the foundational forces that shape health, then, takes humility. It is humility that helps us recognize that sometimes the most important tasks are the least glamorous, the least likely to yield a quick triumph. While the Covid-19 vaccine was developed with remarkable speed, addressing the conditions that allowed Covid-19 to emerge is a long-term project. It will take sustained, multisector engagement with the full range of forces that shape health, not just the ones that garner headlines.

We engaged with these forces during the pandemic because the virus necessitated humility. It showed that it was very clearly in charge and that if we wanted to have healthy lives, we needed to acknowledge our smallness in the face of larger forces. This allowed us to put aside our hubris and be productive. It did not matter whether the task at hand was large or small, whether it involved the latest technology or simply neighbors helping neighbors. We did whatever appeared necessary to navigate the crisis. The same goes for the political leaders who, despite the usual partisan battles, did manage to come together during Covid-19 to provide some economic support to Americans in need.

All this is to the good, and reflects the embrace of humility that facing disaster urges.

Now, however, the winter of our discontent has given way to a time of celebration and possibility. It is up to us to determine whether this moment will be the prologue to an even greater crisis or will lead to a time of unprecedented, historic improvements in health. Vaccines may have ended the pandemic, but the solutions we turned to during the crisis were overwhelmingly based on the intersection of health and the socioeconomic forces that shape our lives. We engaged with the economic drivers of poor health, we took care of each other at the community level, we began a conversation about racial injustice, and, perhaps most important of all, we acknowledged that health is a public good, sustained through collective effort. Such actions can, if we let them, serve as the start of a new approach to health, one based on shoring up the foundations of what truly keeps us well. We need the humility to recognize we must continue to engage with these forces, that our science alone will not be enough to protect us from the contagion next time.

This is particularly important given the potential of hubris to distract our focus from what matters most to health. The risk of backsliding on health is real. Humans have a tendency, when they feel they are out of the woods, to misplace the lessons of hard experience. It would be entirely within our nature to forget what worked during the pandemic and only adopt those solutions again when the next contagion inevitably hits. It is tempting to think we have established a template for navigating pandemics; while this template was not able to prevent mass death during Covid-19, it was able to prevent something resembling the end of the world, and when all is said and done, is that not enough? The trouble is that it was only "enough" for Covid-19 (setting aside, for the moment, how our approach nevertheless failed the thousands who did sicken and die from the virus). It may not, and likely will not, be enough to mitigate the worst of the next pandemic, much less to stop it from happening. Our focus on healthcare has long distracted us from engaging with the conditions that shape health. Not only has it distracted us, but it has made us regard improving these conditions as solutions of a somewhat lower order than those generated by the exciting world of cutting-edge science. "Yes," we might say, "we certainly need better housing, a fairer economy, education for all, and so on. But we have always needed these—such solutions are obvious, old hat. Why should we pursue them when we could pour our money into curing aging or using genetics to design humans who never get sick?"

Such thinking is more than misguided: it is positively dangerous when it causes us to walk back the steps we have taken toward creating a world that is free from contagion. We should have the humility to resist this backsliding and instead engage with the fundamentals of health—in our policies and in our public conversation. To change the world, we must first acknowledge that it is far bigger than we are, that the forces that shape it are more influential than even the best science. It is then our task to work, collectively, toward the solutions we began to advance while the pandemic was still raging. We have a clear choice in this post-pandemic moment. We can yield to the temptation of hubris, ignoring what matters most for health in favor of an approach that opened the door to Covid-19. Or we can have the humility to engage with larger forces, to be aware that we do not know what we do not know, and to advance a vision for health we can see only when we have taken our eye off distractions, however shiny and cutting-edge they may be. How we choose will determine how healthy we are able to be in the years to come.

Epilogue

Covid-19 was not just a virus. It was a story: of our collective health, our vulnerability, and our resilience. This overarching narrative emerged from many smaller narratives. There was the political narrative of the pandemic, the story of governments working to respond to an unprecedented threat. There was the economic narrative, lived across a variety of scales, from multinational corporations scrambling to adapt to changing workplace realities to the dinner tables around which many people, newly unemployed, worked out monthly expenses. It was a global story, as an epidemic that started in China crossed provincial and then international borders to engulf the world. At a deeper level, it was the story of individuals, each trying to navigate the difficulties of the moment. The sick and the well, those who recovered from the disease and those who succumbed to it. And just as the broader narrative of Covid-19 is anchored in these individual stories, each of these stories has something to say about the foundational forces that shaped the arc of the pandemic.

The aim of this book has been to take you, the reader, on a journey through these foundational forces. At core, these forces are the world we live in, the conditions that create health, the values that should inform these conditions, and the science that can help improve our understanding of these conditions. I realize that these forces may be an unexpected focus for a book like this. More expected would have been a book about the science of disease transmission and the research areas that generated the Covid-19 vaccines. Instead, we have spent twelve chapters discussing something with which we are all familiar: the context of our lives. I will be the first to admit there is nothing particularly new here (recognizing that this is a slightly heretical admission for an author to make). In discussing the forces that shape health, I am discussing conditions with which we interact each day, and which shape our lives at every moment. Precisely because these conditions are so familiar, we do not always think of them, and we certainly do not always think of their relationship to our health. Covid-19 changed this, laying bare these foundational forces and how our health is shaped by the role they play in our society and in our lives. Health does not depend on any single factor; rather, it depends on a range of intersecting conditions. The pandemic showed the importance of engaging with this dynamic, of addressing the drivers of health, as a means of preventing disease.

This understanding came to us, sadly, through pain and suffering. Earlier in the book, I referred to Robert Kennedy's speech after the murder of Martin Luther King Jr. During that speech, Kennedy quoted from the ancient Greek playwright Aeschylus. He said:

> My favorite poet was Aeschylus. And he once wrote: "Even in our sleep, pain which cannot forget falls drop by drop upon the heart until, in our own despair, against our will, comes wisdom through the awful grace of God."

During Covid-19, we experienced the truth of these words. The pain of that moment generated the wisdom to understand the forces that truly shape health. Yet there is no guarantee that this will prove to be "pain which cannot forget." Many of us, with good reason, would like nothing more than to forget Covid-19. The danger, as I have argued, of this post-pandemic moment is that as memory of the crisis fades, our understanding of its causes will also fade. This book is, in part, an effort to keep the conditions that matter most to health at the top of our minds and at the center of the public conversation. It is an effort to keep our hard-won wisdom intact. It would be a shame if, after all we went through, we found ourselves back where we started in our approach to health. It would also be dangerous. It would be missing a chance to create the healthier world that is our best defense against the contagion next time. It would be to invite catastrophe: a recurrence of the status quo that left us vulnerable to disease.

Covid-19 exposed the extent to which this status quo has poorly served us. During the pandemic, we saw how the inequalities present in our society create cracks in the foundations of health, making these foundations unsound. These cracks include economic disadvantage, lack of care for older adults, disparities in housing, and the legacy of racial injustice. I have given particular focus in this book to the challenge of race, reflecting the scope of its influence on health in the United States and the fact that for much of our history the effect of racial injustice on health was simply not addressed at the level it should have been. Our failures on race have been a constant challenge for health in this country—most acutely for the health of communities of color, but, ultimately, for the health of everyone. The pandemic amply demonstrated that when we allow the health of any group to languish, we are creating the conditions for our own sickness. This is why care for the marginalized, the vulnerable, and the dispossessed should be at the heart of our approach to health in the post-pandemic world.

Our failure to pursue this approach before Covid-19 reflects our broader failure to see health as a public good. When we regard health as purely a matter of medicine and treatments, when we see it as a commodity we can purchase rather than as a public good everyone can access and which we sustain through collective investment, we have created a world where it is easy for the health of certain groups to slip through the cracks. Supporting the health of these groups depends on our willingness to see their health as inextricably linked to our own, and to realize that this connection necessitates approaching health as a public good. From the very beginning, Covid-19 showed us how closely linked our health really is, that none of us can be healthy unless we are all healthy. Ensuring we can all be healthy means embracing a perspective that sees health as a public good.

Preventing the contagion next time, then, rests on understanding that health is a product of foundational forces, that it is a public good, and that addressing it as a public good means recognizing the connections that bind our health together and taking special care to support the health of the marginalized. The stakes of getting this right could not be higher. The damage done by Covid-19 did not just reflect the characteristics of a novel virus, it reflected the characteristics of a society with a misguided approach to health. This approach opened the door to widespread preventable sickness and death. By allowing itself to be marked by socioeconomic divides, by choosing to see health as a commodity, by investing in doctors and medicines at the expense of health, the United States set itself up to fail during a crisis such as Covid-19.

And Covid-19 was a summer holiday compared to what could come next. The contagion next time could take any form, target any group. It behooves us, then, to build a world where everyone can be healthy. Ultimately, being prepared means choosing health. It means saying that health is the highest possible good, then acting, collectively, like we mean it. This requires a reorientation of our social, economic, and political priorities, and accepting the trade-offs this would entail. This may feel uncomfortable at first, as it will mean trading a simpler view of health for one that engages with the full complexity of what matters most for our collective well-being. However, this trade-off is essential for building a healthier world, one that is no longer threatened by pandemics. It is understandable that we might resist the dramatic changes necessary to create such a world. But another lesson of Covid-19 is that the world changes on its own, whether we like it or not. Accepting that dramatic changes are inevitable, we should take care that they are changes that benefit health.

We have already taken steps in this direction. Many of the actions we embraced in order to deal with the emergency of Covid-19—from economic support that would buffer some of the effects of the recession to efforts to provide relief for marginalized groups—could well serve as the foundation for the future we need, if only we choose to see them this way. This starts with recognizing that the need they addressed—the deep-rootedness of poor health in this country—did not dissipate with the end of Covid-19. From opioids and mental illness to obesity, gun violence, poverty, racism, corporate practices that harm health, and the bad policy that sustains these challenges, there remains no shortage of preventable conditions that sicken and kill scores of Americans each year. And there is no reason we cannot address these challenges with the same ingenuity, ambition, and collective effort we applied to Covid-19.

Fundamentally, we need to choose health, recognizing that choosing health means not just creating better drugs but also accepting responsibility for creating a healthier world. During Covid-19, we chose health—individually, in our households, among our extended families and friend groups, in our towns, in our cities. We recognized that health is possible only when we all work for it, and so we did, striving toward the healthiest possible world, even in the midst of sickness and death. When governments and corporations chose to place health at the heart of their endeavors during the pandemic, their actions were informed by the fact that we had already made this choice for ourselves at the grassroots level.

This reflects another lesson of Covid-19: we do not have to wait for the leadership of the federal government and international organizations to choose health. Certainly, aligning these bodies with health should be our ultimate goal—we need the captain of our ship, the crew, and the course we chart all aiming in the direction of better health. However, the pandemic has shown how neighborhoods, towns, and cities can take the lead in shifting paradigms. In 2020, facing global challenge, we saw how the world is smaller than we often think it is. We can use this perspective to our advantage, leveraging our connections toward the collective pursuit of better health, a pursuit we embraced during Covid-19 with new dedication and purpose. There were shortcomings and missed opportunities, yes, but the overwhelming takeaway of what we have been through is that when we value health and feel it is truly at stake, there are no limits to what we can do. We need to apply this lesson, while we can, to the work that is so clearly cut out for us in the wake of Covid-19.

I chose to call this book *The Contagion Next Time* in homage to James Baldwin's book *The Fire Next Time*. In his book, Baldwin engages with the issue of race in America and how we need to think differently about this subject in order to create a better society. This book argues for a similar change in perspective around health. It also recognizes the ineluctable role that reckoning with race has to play in America if we are to create a better, healthier country. If we are to prevent the next pandemic, we need to engage with the forces that shape health to create a world that is resistant to contagion. We need to stop prioritizing medicine over the core drivers of health and start addressing deep-seated racial and socioeconomic injustices. Absent this change, we risk seeing not merely a repeat of Covid-19 but an amplification of it, in the form of a contagion from which we may not collectively be able to recover.

Like the ship metaphor with which I began this book, the title of *The Fire Next Time* refers to a storm—a flood. Baldwin borrowed the phrase from the lyrics of a spiritual that includes the lines "God gave Noah the rainbow sign / No more water, the fire next time." This warns us to be prepared, that the recent crisis could serve as prologue to an even more difficult future if we do not take steps to address the failure and injustices that create the conditions for catastrophe.

We have just been through a storm. We are understandably tired, and relieved to put this trauma behind us. The last possibility we wish to face is that of something worse on the horizon. But it is an uncomfortable fact that the dynamics that led to the Covid-19 pandemic are still in place. Fortunately, these dynamics are accompanied by something new: the wisdom that comes from adversity. Our experience of the pandemic showed us the way toward a healthier world. This book is an effort to organize and explain what Covid-19 taught us, to inform a conversation that leads to the changes we need to make before the next contagion. It is now up to us to heed the lessons of a difficult moment and do what must be done while the seas are still calm, the sun still visible in the sky.

References

EPIGRAPH

Camus A. *The Plague*. New York: Knopf Doubleday; 2012.

Dhliwayo M. Goodreads website. https://www.goodreads.com/quotes/8169571-you-don-t-command-wind-in-the-direction-it-blows-but. Accessed January 13, 2021.

INTRODUCTION

Cyranoski D. Bat Cave Solves Mystery of Deadly SARS Virus—and Suggests New Outbreak Could Occur. *Nature*. 2017; 552: 15–16.

SARS Basics Fact Sheet. Centers for Disease Control and Prevention website. https://www.cdc.gov/sars/about/fs-sars.html. Updated December 6, 2017. Accessed December 30, 2020.

Hawryluck L, Gold WL, Robinson S, Pogorski S, Galea S, Styra R. SARS Control and Psychological Effects of Quarantine, Toronto, Canada. *Emerging Infectious Diseases*. 2004; 10(7): 1206–1212.

CDC SARS Response Timeline. Centers for Disease Control and Prevention website. https://www.cdc.gov/about/history/sars/timeline.htm. Updated April 26, 2013. Accessed December 30, 2020.

Frequently Asked Questions About SARS. Centers for Disease Control and Prevention website. https://www.cdc.gov/sars/about/faq.html. Updated May 3, 2005. Accessed December 30, 2020.

Coronavirus Cases. Worldometer website. https://www.worldometers.info/coronavirus/coronavirus-cases/. Updated December 30, 2020. Accessed December 30, 2020.

Nackerdien Z. Viral Load Peaks in First Week of COVID-19 Symptom Onset. *MedPage Today*. https://www.medpagetoday.org/infectiousdisease/covid19/90035?vpass=1. Accessed December 30, 2020.

Seladi-Schulman J, medically reviewed by Goodwin M. COVID-19 vs. SARS: How Do They Differ? Healthline website. https://www.healthline.com/health/coronavirus-vs-sars. Published April 2, 2020. Accessed December 30, 2020.

Schwartz ND, Casselman B, Koeze E. How Bad Is Unemployment? "Literally Off the Charts." *The New York Times.* May 8, 2020. https://www.nytimes.com/interactive/2020/05/08/business/economy/april-jobs-report.html. Accessed December 30, 2020.

Hill E, Tiefenthäler A, Triebert C, Jordan D, Willis H, Stein R. How George Floyd Was Killed in Police Custody. *The New York Times.* May 31, 2020. https://www.nytimes.com/2020/05/31/us/george-floyd-investigation.html. Accessed December 30, 2020.

Keshavan M. "The Direct Result of Racism": Covid-19 Lays Bare How Discrimination Drives Health Disparities Among Black People. *STAT News.* June 9, 2020. https://www.statnews.com/2020/06/09/systemic-racism-black-health-disparities/. Accessed December 30, 2020.

Williams DR, Collins C. Racial Residential Segregation: A Fundamental Cause of Racial Disparities in Health. *Public Health Reports.* 2001; 116(5): 404–416.

Blankenship KM, Del Rio Gonzalez AM, Keene DE, Groves AK, Rosenberg AP. Mass Incarceration, Race Inequality, and Health: Expanding Concepts and Assessing Impacts on Well-being. *Social Science & Medicine.* 2018; 215: 45–52.

Flanders-Stepans MB. Alarming Racial Differences in Maternal Mortality. *The Journal of Perinatal Education.* 2000; 9(2): 50–51.

Chetty R, et al. The Association Between Income and Life Expectancy in the United States, 2001–2014. *JAMA: The Journal of the American Medical Association.* 2016; 315(16): 1750–1766.

Time. May 15, 2017 issue. https://time.com/magazine/us/4766607/may-15th-2017-vol-189-no-18-u-s/. Accessed December 30, 2020.

CHAPTER 1. A BETTER AND HEALTHIER TIME TO BE ALIVE THAN EVER

Sumner A, Hoy C, Ortiz-Juarez E. Estimates of the Impact of COVID-19 on Global Poverty. WIDER Working Paper 2020/43. Helsinki: UNU-WIDER; 2020.

Press Release: COVID-19 Fallout Could Push Half a Billion People into Poverty in Developing Countries. United Nations University World Institute for Development Economics Research website. https://www.wider.unu.edu/news/press-release-covid-19-fallout-could-push-half-billion-people-poverty-developing-countries. Published April 8, 2020. Accessed December 31, 2020.

Roser M, Ortiz-Ospina E. Global Education. Our World in Data website. https://ourworldindata.org/global-education. Published 2016. Accessed December 31, 2020.

Fauci AS, Lane HC. Four Decades of HIV/AIDS—Much Accomplished, Much to Do. *The New England Journal of Medicine.* 2020; 383(1): 1–4.

The Editors of Encyclopaedia Britannica. Buggy. Encyclopaedia Britannica website. https://www.britannica.com/technology/buggy. Accessed December 31, 2020.

National Center for Health Statistics. Health, United States, 2010: With Special Feature on Death and Dying. 2011. Centers for Disease Control and Prevention website. https://www.cdc.gov/nchs/data/hus/hus10.pdf. Accessed December 31, 2020.

Life Expectancy. Centers for Disease Control and Prevention website. https://www.cdc.gov/nchs/fastats/life-expectancy.htm. Updated October 30, 2020. Accessed December 31, 2020.

Baicus A. History of Polio Vaccination. *World Journal of Virology*. 2012; 1(4): 108–114.

Urbanization. Encyclopedia.com website. https://www.encyclopedia.com/defense/energy-government-and-defense-magazines/urbanization. Updated December 20, 2020. Accessed December 31, 2020.

History.com Editors. US Immigration Before 1965. History website. https://www.history.com/topics/immigration/u-s-immigration-before-1965. Published October 29, 2009. Updated July 28, 2020. Accessed December 31, 2020.

Arbuckle AQ. 2016. How the Other Half Lives. Mashable website. https://mashable.com/2016/04/13/new york tenement photos/. Accessed December 31, 2020.

History.com Editors. Child Labor. History website. https://www.history.com/topics/industrial-revolution/child-labor. Published October 27, 2009. Updated April 17, 2020. Accessed December 31, 2020.

Sherman E. 25 Haunting Photos of Life Inside New York's Tenements. All That's Interesting website. https://allthatsinteresting.com/tenement-new-york-photos-facts#6. Published May 29, 2016. Updated June 22, 2020. Accessed December 31, 2020.

Roser M, Ortiz-Ospina E, Ritchie H. Life Expectancy. Our World in Data website. https://ourworldindata.org/life-expectancy. Published 2013. Updated October 2019. Accessed December 31, 2020.

World Population Living in Extreme Poverty, 1820–2015. Our World in Data website. https://ourworldindata.org/grapher/world-population-in-extreme-poverty-absolute. Accessed December 31, 2020.

Rutstein D. Multidimensional Child Poverty in Sub-Saharan Africa. UNICEF Connect website. https://blogs.unicef.org/blog/multidimensional-child-poverty-in-sub-saharan-africa/. Published January 27, 2015. Accessed December 31, 2020.

Child Poverty. UNICEF website. https://www.unicef.org/social-policy/child-poverty. Accessed December 31, 2020.

Roser M, Ritchie H. Hunger and Undernourishment. Our World in Data website. https://ourworldindata.org/hunger-and-undernourishment. Accessed December 31, 2020.

Roser M, Ritchie H, Dadonaite B. Child and Infant Mortality. Our World in Data website. https://ourworldindata.org/child-mortality. Published 2013. Updated November 2019. Accessed December 31, 2020.

The Editors of Encyclopaedia Britannica. Little Nell. Encyclopaedia Britannica website. https://www.britannica.com/topic/Little-Nell-fictional-character. Accessed December 31, 2020.

Roser M. Measurement Matters—The Decline of Maternal Mortality. Our World in Data website. https://ourworldindata.org/measurement-matters-the-decline-of-maternal-mortality. Published October 25, 2017. Accessed December 31, 2020.

Children Born per Woman, 1810. Our World in Data website. https://our worldindata.org/grapher/children-born-per-woman?year=1810. Accessed December 31, 2020.

Martin E. Money Is Flooding into These 10 Industries That Are Adding Jobs and Thriving. CNBC. October 16, 2018. https://www.cnbc.com/2018/10/16/top-10-industries-that-are-hiring-thriving-and-making-money.html. Accessed December 31, 2020.

Galea S. *Well: What We Need to Talk About When We Talk About Health.* New York: Oxford University Press; 2019.

Roser M, Ritchie H. Maternal Mortality. Our World in Data website. https://ourworldindata.org/maternal-mortality. Accessed January 11, 2020.

Health Spending (Indicator). OECD Data website. https://data.oecd.org/healthres/health-spending.htm. Accessed January 11, 2020.

Number of Deaths by Risk Factor for Under-5s, World, 2017. Our World in Data website. https://ourworldindata.org/grapher/deaths-by-risk-under5s. Accessed January 11, 2020.

CHAPTER 2. AN UNHEALTHY COUNTRY

Hobbes M. Will America Let COVID-19 Become the Next HIV? *HuffPost.* August 11, 2020. https://www.huffpost.com/entry/will-america-let-covid-19-become-next-hiv_n_5f31ad0ec5b6960c066af7d1?guccounter=1. Accessed January 2, 2021.

Chetty R, et al. The Association Between Income and Life Expectancy in the United States, 2001–2014. *JAMA: The Journal of the American Medical Association.* 2016; 315(16): 1750–1766.

Acri MC, et al. The Intersection of Extreme Poverty and Familial Mental Health in the United States. *Social Work in Mental Health.* 2017; 15(6):677–689.

Shaw KM, Theis KA, Self-Brown S, Roblin DW, Barker L. Chronic Disease Disparities by County Economic Status and Metropolitan Classification, Behavioral Risk Factor Surveillance System, 2013. *Preventing Chronic Disease.* 2016; 13: 160088.

Equity of Opportunity. US Department of Education website. https://www.ed.gov/equity. Accessed January 2, 2021.

Galea S. A Good Education—The Best Prevention? Boston University School of Public Health website. https://www.bu.edu/sph/news/articles/2016/a-good-education-the-best-prevention/. Published May 8, 2016. Accessed January 2, 2021.

Poverty. Healthy People website. https://www.healthypeople.gov/2020/topics-objectives/topic/social-determinants-health/interventions-resources/poverty. Accessed January 2, 2021.

NCI Staff. African American Men More Likely to Die from Low-Grade Prostate Cancer. National Cancer Institute website. https://www.cancer.gov/news-events/cancer-currents-blog/2019/prostate-cancer-death-disparities-black-men. Published January 28, 2019. Accessed January 2, 2021.

African American Women and Breast Cancer. Breast Cancer Prevention Partners website. https://www.bcpp.org/resource/african-american-women-and-breast-cancer/. Accessed January 2, 2021.

Hispanic Health. Centers for Disease Control and Prevention website. https://www.cdc.gov/vitalsigns/hispanic-health/index.html. Accessed January 2, 2021.

Reagan R. Inaugural Address. January 20, 1981. Avalon Project website. https://avalon.law.yale.edu/20th_century/reagan1.asp. Accessed January 2, 2021.

Hofstede D. California Cowboy Ronald Reagan Acted the Part and Lived It Too. Cowboys & Indians. June 26, 2020. https://www.cowboysindians.com/2020/06/reagan-on-the-range/. Accessed January 2, 2021.

Ronald Reagan on Big Government | Most Terrifying Words. Reagan.com website. https://www.reagan.com/ronald-reagan-on-big-government-most-terrifying-words. Published August 17, 2018. Accessed January 2, 2021.

Silver C. The Top 25 Economies in the World. Investopedia website. https://www.investopedia.com/insights/worlds-top-economies/. Updated December 24, 2020. Accessed January 2, 2021.

Newman K. US Life Expectancy Falls as Drug Overdoses, Suicides Rise. *US News & World Report*. November 29, 2018. https://www.usnews.com/news/healthiest-communities/articles/2018-11-29/us-life-expectancy-falls-as-drug-overdoses-suicides-rise. Accessed January 2, 2021.

Galea S. The Real Reason Why American Lives Are Getting Shorter. *HuffPost*. December 7, 2018. https://www.huffpost.com/entry/opinion-life-expectancy-americans_n_5c0982b0e4b0b6cdaf5d37c8. Accessed January 2, 2021.

Rappleye E. US Life Expectancy Faces Longest Decline Since WWI, Spanish Flu Pandemic. *Becker's Hospital Review*. July 9, 2019. https://www.beckershospitalreview.com/care-coordination/us-life-expectancy-faces-longest-decline-since-wwi-spanish-flu-pandemic.html. Accessed January 2, 2021.

Faust JS, Lin Z, del Rio C. Comparison of Estimated Excess Deaths in New York City During the COVID-19 and 1918 Influenza Pandemics. *JAMA Network Open*. 2020; 3(8): e2017527.

Overdose Death Rates. National Institute on Drug Abuse website. https://www.drugabuse.gov/drug-topics/trends-statistics/overdose-death-rates. Accessed January 2, 2021.

Serletis G. Deadly High-Purity Fentanyl from China Is Entering the US Through E-Commerce Channels. US International Trade Commission Executive Briefings on Trade, September 2019. US International Trade Commission website. https://www.usitc.gov/publications/332/executive_briefings/ebot_george_serletis_fentanyl_from_china_pdf.pdf. Accessed January 2, 2021.

Suicide Statistics. American Foundation for Suicide Prevention website. https://afsp.org/suicide-statistics/. Accessed January 2, 2021.

Suicide Facts & Figures: United States 2020. Flyer from American Foundation for Suicide Prevention. https://www.datocms-assets.com/12810/1587128056-usfactsfiguresflyer-2.pdf. Accessed January 2, 2021.

Ettman CK, Gradus JL, Galea S. Invited Commentary: Reckoning with the Relationship Between Stressors and Suicide Attempts in a Time of COVID-19. *American Journal of Epidemiology.* 2020; 189(11): 1275–1277.

Heart Disease Facts. Centers for Disease Control and Prevention website. https://www.cdc.gov/heartdisease/facts.htm. Accessed January 2, 2021.

US Cancer Statistics Working Group. US Cancer Statistics Data Visualizations Tool, based on 2019 submission data (1999–2017): US Department of Health and Human Services, Centers for Disease Control and Prevention and National Cancer Institute. Centers for Disease Control and Prevention website. www.cdc.gov/cancer/dataviz. Released June 2020. Accessed January 2, 2021.

Asthma Facts and Figures. Asthma and Allergy Foundation of America website. https://www.aafa.org/asthma-facts/. Updated June 2019. Accessed January 2, 2021.

Adult Obesity Facts. Centers for Disease Control and Prevention website. https://www.cdc.gov/obesity/data/adult.html. Accessed January 2, 2021.

People with Certain Medical Conditions. Centers for Disease Control and Prevention website. https://www.cdc.gov/coronavirus/2019-ncov/need-extra-precautions/people-with-medical-conditions.html. Updated December 29, 2020. Accessed January 2, 2021.

Larger Portion Sizes Contribute to US Obesity Problem. National Heart, Lung, and Blood Institute website. https://www.nhlbi.nih.gov/health/educational/wecan/news-events/matte1.htm. Updated February 13, 2013. Accessed January 2, 2021.

Curley B. How to Combat "Food Deserts" and "Food Swamps." Healthline website. https://www.healthline.com/health-news/combat-food-deserts-and-food-swamps#1. Updated September 24, 2018. Accessed January 2, 2021.

Getz L. Food Deserts: Where Healthy Options Are Only a Mirage. *Today's Dietitian.* October 2008. https://www.todaysdietitian.com/newarchives/092208p48.shtml. Accessed January 2, 2021.

Inequity. Merriam-Webster website. https://www.merriam-webster.com/dictionary/inequity. Accessed January 3, 2021.

Robinson NJ. Slavery Was Very Recent. *Current Affairs*. October 20, 2016. https://www.currentaffairs.org/2016/10/slavery-was-very-recent. Accessed January 3, 2021.

Lincoln A. Lincoln's Second Inaugural Address. March 4, 1865. National Park Service website. https://www.nps.gov/linc/learn/historyculture/lincoln-second-inaugural.htm. Accessed January 3, 2021.

Bromwich D. Lincoln as Realist and Revolutionist. Neubauer Collegium Director's Lecture, given at the Neubauer Collegium for Culture and Society, University of Chicago, February 11, 2016. YouTube. https://www.youtube.com/watch?v=-ZN6qdQ6nnU. Accessed January 3, 2021.

Reeves RV, Matthew DB. 6 Charts Showing Race Gaps Within the American Middle Class. Brookings Institution website. https://www.brookings.edu/blog/social-mobility-memos/2016/10/21/6-charts-showing-race-gaps-within-the-american-middle-class/. Published October 21, 2016. Accessed January 3, 2021.

Matthew DB, Rodrigue E, Reeves RV. Time for Justice: Tackling Race Inequalities in Health and Housing. Brookings Institution website. https://www.brookings.edu/research/time-for-justice-tackling-race-inequalities-in-health-and-housing/#_edn8. Published October 19, 2016. Accessed January 3, 2021.

Szabo L, Recht H. The Other COVID Risks: How Race, Income, ZIP Code Influence Who Lives or Dies. *Kaiser Health News*. April 22, 2020. https://khn.org/news/covid-south-other-risk-factors-how-race-income-zip-code-influence-who-lives-or-dies/. Accessed January 3, 2021.

Nave RL. Mississippi Still Has Worst Poverty, Household Income. *Mississippi Today*. September 14, 2017. https://mississippitoday.org/2017/09/14/mississippi-still-worst-poverty-household-income-u-s/. Accessed January 3, 2021.

Knueven L. The Typical American Household Earns $61,000 a Year. Here Are 15 States Where the Typical Resident Earns Even Less. *Business Insider*. August 19, 2019. https://www.businessinsider.com/personal-finance/poorest-states-in-the-us-by-median-household-income-2019-8. Accessed January 3, 2021.

The Burden of Diabetes in Mississippi. American Diabetes Association website. http://main.diabetes.org/dorg/PDFs/Advocacy/burden-of-diabetes/mississippi.pdf. Accessed January 3, 2021.

Asthma and African Americans. US Department of Health and Human Services Office of Minority Health website. https://minorityhealth.hhs.gov/omh/browse.aspx?lvl=4&lvlid=15. Updated January 9, 2018. Accessed January 3, 2021.

National Center for Health Statistics. Health, United States, 2017: With Special Feature on Mortality. 2018. Centers for Disease Control and Prevention website. https://www.cdc.gov/nchs/data/hus/hus17.pdf. Accessed January 11, 2021.

APM Research Lab Staff. The Color of Coronavirus: Covid-19 Deaths by Race and Ethnicity in the US. APM Research Lab website. https://www.apmresearchlab.org/covid/deaths-by-race. Accessed January 11, 2021.

Kamal R. How Does US Life Expectancy Compare to Other Countries? Peterson-KFF Health System Tracker website. https://www.healthsystemtracker.org/chart-collection/u-s-life-expectancy-compare-countries/#item-start. Published December 23, 2019. Accessed January 11, 2021.

World Health Organization. United States of America. In: World Health Organization—Noncommunicable Diseases (NCD) Country Profiles, 2018. https://www.who.int/nmh/countries/usa_en.pdf?ua=1. Accessed January 11, 2021.

CHAPTER 3. AN UNHEALTHY WORLD

Galea S. The Unnecessary Persistence of Tuberculosis. *HuffPost*. October 26, 2016. https://www.huffpost.com/entry/the-unnecessary-persisten_b_12661768. Accessed January 9, 2021.

Tuberculosis. World Health Organization website. https://www.who.int/news-room/fact-sheets/detail/tuberculosis. Accessed January 9, 2021.

Thomas N. Updated CDC Guidance Acknowledges Coronavirus Can Spread Through the Air. CNN. September 20, 2020. https://www.cnn.com/2020/09/20/health/cdc-coronavirus-airborne-transmission/index.html. Accessed January 9, 2021.

US Department of Health and Human Services, Centers for Disease Control and Prevention National Center for HIV/AIDS, Viral Hepatitis, STD, and TB Prevention, Division of Tuberculosis Elimination. Questions and Answers About Tuberculosis (TB). 2014. Centers for Disease Control and Prevention website. https://www.cdc.gov/tb/publications/faqs/pdfs/qa.pdf. Accessed January 9, 2021.

Horsburgh Jr CR, Barry III CE, Lange C. Treatment of Tuberculosis. *The New England Journal of Medicine*. 2015; 373: 2149–2160.

Lawler D. Some Countries Are Hardly Testing for COVID-19 at All. *Axios*. May 23, 2020. https://www.axios.com/poor-countries-coronavirus-testing-d60610b5-52c4-4a42-96ce-4f603bd8bcec.html. Accessed January 9, 2021.

Kramer S. More Americans Say They Are Regularly Wearing Masks in Stores and Other Businesses. Pew Research Center website. https://www.pewresearch.org/fact-tank/2020/08/27/more-americans-say-they-are-regularly-wearing-masks-in-stores-and-other-businesses/. Published August 27, 2020. Accessed January 9, 2021.

Chaisson RE, Martinson NA. Tuberculosis in Africa—Combating an HIV-Driven Crisis. *The New England Journal of Medicine*. 2008; 358: 1089–1092.

World Health Organization. WHO Report on the Global Tobacco Epidemic, 2008: The MPOWER Package. 2008. World Health Organization website. https://www.who.int/tobacco/mpower/2008/en/. Accessed January 9, 2021.

Pesce G, et al. Time and Age Trends in Smoking Cessation in Europe. *PLOS One*. 2019; 14(2): e0211976.

American Heart Association News. Smoking in America: Why More Americans Are Kicking the Habit. American Heart Association website. https://www.heart.org/en/news/2018/08/29/smoking-in-america-why-more-americans-are-kicking-the-habit. Published August 30, 2018. Accessed January 9, 2021.

The Toll of Tobacco Around the World. Campaign for Tobacco-Free Kids website. https://www.tobaccofreekids.org/problem/toll-global. Updated June 18, 2020. Accessed January 9, 2021.

World Health Organization. WHO Report on the Global Tobacco Epidemic, 2011: Warning About the Dangers of Tobacco. 2008. World Health Organization website. https://www.who.int/tobacco/global_report/2011/en/. Accessed January 9, 2021.

Children: Improving Survival and Well-Being. World Health Organization website. https://www.who.int/news-room/fact-sheets/detail/children-reducing-mortality. Accessed January 9, 2021.

Cardiovascular Diseases. World Health Organization website. https://www.who.int/health-topics/cardiovascular-diseases/#tab=tab_1. Accessed January 9, 2021.

Global Cancer Facts & Figures. American Cancer Society website. https://www.cancer.org/research/cancer-facts-statistics/global.html. Accessed January 9, 2021.

Nishiga M, Wang DW, Han Y, Lewis DB, Wu JC. COVID-19 and Cardiovascular Disease: From Basic Mechanisms to Clinical Perspectives. *Nature Reviews Cardiology*. 2020; 17(9): 543–558.

Common Questions About the COVID-19 Outbreak. American Cancer Society website. https://www.cancer.org/latest-news/common-questions-about-the-new-coronavirus-outbreak.html. Accessed January 10, 2021.

Air Pollution. World Health Organization website. https://www.who.int/health-topics/air-pollution#tab=tab_1. Accessed January 10, 2021.

Ambient Air Pollution. World Health Organization website. https://www.who.int/teams/environment-climate-change-and-health/air-quality-and-health/ambient-air-pollution. Accessed January 10, 2021.

Katz C. People in Poor Neighborhoods Breathe More Hazardous Particles. *Scientific American*. November 1, 2012. https://www.scientificamerican.com/article/people-poor-neighborhoods-breate-more-hazardous-particles/. Accessed January 10, 2021.

Gupta A, et al. Air Pollution Aggravating COVID-19 Lethality? Exploration in Asian Cities Using Statistical Models. *Environment, Development and Sustainability*. 2020.

The Visual and Data Journalism Team. California and Oregon 2020 Wildfires in Maps, Graphics and Images. BBC News. September 17, 2020. https://www .bbc.com/news/world-us-canada-54180049. Accessed January 10, 2021.

Duginski P. How Smoke from California Wildfires Turns the Sky Red. *Los Angeles Times*. September 15, 2020. https://www.latimes.com/california/ story/2020-09-15/how-california-wildfire-smoke-turns-sky-red. Accessed January 10, 2021.

Selsky A. Lightning Storm, Easterly Wind: How the Wildfires Got So Bad. *Associated Press*. September 17, 2020. https://apnews.com/article/salem-storms-oregon-forestry-weather-2b305e6af052e6fe1d4bc247804ef569. Accessed January 10, 2021.

Temple J. Suppressing Fires Has Failed. Here's What California Needs to Do Instead. *MIT Technology Review*. September 17, 2020. https://www.tech nologyreview.com/2020/09/17/1008473/wildfires-california-prescribed-burns-climate-change-forests/. Accessed January 10, 2021.

Shultz JM, Fugate C, Galea S. Cascading Risks of COVID-19 Resurgence During an Active 2020 Atlantic Hurricane Season. *JAMA: The Journal of the American Medical Association*. 324(10): 935–936.

The Universal Declaration of Human Rights. The United Nations website. http://www.un.org/en/universal-declaration-human-rights/. Accessed January 10, 2021.

Galea S. Climate Change Is Making Us Sick. *Cognoscenti*. WBUR. June 2, 2017. https://www.wbur.org/cognoscenti/2017/06/02/climate-change-is-making-us-sick. Accessed January 10, 2021.

Galea S. By Cutting Ties with the World Health Organization, Trump Endangers Global Public Health. *STAT News*. May 31, 2020. https://www .statnews.com/2020/05/31/cutting-ties-with-world-health-organization-endangers-global-public-health/. Accessed January 10, 2021.

Family Separation Under the Trump Administration—a Timeline. Southern Poverty Law Center website. https://www.splcenter.org/news/2020/06/ 17/family-separation-under-trump-administration-timeline. Published June 17, 2020. Accessed January 10, 2021.

Ritchie H, Roser M. Urbanization. Our World in Data website. https:// ourworldindata.org/urbanization. Published September 2018. Updated November 2019. Accessed January 10, 2021.

Death Rate from Tuberculosis, 2017. Our World in Data website. https:// ourworldindata.org/grapher/tuberculosis-death-rates. Accessed January 11, 2021.

Ritchie H, Roser M. Smoking. Our World in Data website. https://our worldindata.org/smoking. Published May 2013. Updated November 2019. Accessed January 11, 2021.

CHAPTER 4. WHO WE ARE: THE FOUNDATIONAL FORCES

Joseph A, illustrations by Reddy M. The Road Ahead: Charting the Coronavirus Pandemic over the Next 12 Months—and Beyond. *STAT News.* September 22, 2020. https://www.statnews.com/feature/coronavi rus/the-road-ahead-the-next-12-months-and-beyond/. Accessed January 9, 2021.

Spellings S, Fass M (Editor). Cloth Masks to Shop Now. *Vogue.* https://www .vogue.com/slideshow/stylish-face-masks-to-shop-now. Accessed January 9, 2021.

Horsley S. 38.6 Million Have Filed for Unemployment Since March. NPR. May 21, 2020. https://www.npr.org/sections/coronavirus-live-updates/ 2020/05/21/859836248/38-6-million-have-filed-for-unemployment- since-march. Accessed January 9, 2021.

Hulse C, Cochrane E. As Coronavirus Spread, Largest Stimulus in History United a Polarized Senate. *The New York Times.* March 26, 2020. https:// www.nytimes.com/2020/03/26/us/coronavirus-senate-stimulus-package .html. Accessed January 9, 2021.

Bernard TS, Lieber R. F.A.Q. on Stimulus Checks, Unemployment and the Coronavirus Plan. *The New York Times.* https://www.nytimes.com/ article/coronavirus-stimulus-package-questions-answers.html. Updated December 23, 2020. Accessed January 9, 2021.

Pethokoukis J. Are We All Milton Keynesians Now? *The Dispatch* (from American Enterprise Institute). February 10, 2020. https://www.aei.org/ articles/are-we-all-milton-keynesians-now/. Accessed January 9, 2021.

The Link Between COVID-19 and CVD. World Heart Federation website. https://www.world-heart-federation.org/covid-19-and-cvd/. Accessed January 9, 2021.

Abdalla SM, Yu S, Galea S. Trends in Cardiovascular Disease Prevalence by Income Level in the United States. *JAMA Network Open.* 2020; 3(9): e2018150.

Galea S. Racism and the Health of the Public. Boston University School of Public Health website. https://www.bu.edu/sph/news/articles/2015/ racism-and-the-health-of-the-public/. Published May 3, 2015. Accessed January 9, 2021.

Paradies Y. A Systematic Review of Empirical Research on Self-Reported Racism and Health. *International Journal of Epidemiology.* 2006; 35(4): 888–901.

Taylor TR, et al. Racial Discrimination and Breast Cancer Incidence in US Black Women: The Black Women's Health Study. *American Journal of Epidemiology.* 2007; 166(1): 46–54.

Ettman CK, Abdalla SM, Cohen GH, Sampson L, Vivier PM, Galea S. Prevalence of Depression Symptoms in US Adults Before and During the COVID-19 Pandemic. *JAMA Network Open.* 2020; 3(9): e2019686.

Plumer B. What Would Happen if the Yellowstone Supervolcano Actually Erupted? *Vox.* December 15, 2014. https://www.vox.com/2014/9/5/6108169/yellowstone-supervolcano-eruption. Accessed January 9, 2021.

Klein N. *The Shock Doctrine: The Rise of Disaster Capitalism.* New York: Picador; 2007.

Solis M. Coronavirus Is the Perfect Disaster for "Disaster Capitalism." *Vice.* March 13, 2020. https://www.vice.com/en/article/5dmqyk/naomi-klein-interview-on-coronavirus-and-disaster-capitalism-shock-doctrine. Accessed January 9, 2021.

Ritchie H, Roser M. Causes of Death. Our World in Data website. https://ourworldindata.org/causes-of-death. Published February 2018. Updated December 2019. Accessed January 11, 2021.

CHAPTER 5. WHERE WE LIVE, WORK, AND PLAY

McLeod S. Maslow's Hierarchy of Needs. Simply Psychology website. https://www.simplypsychology.org/maslow.html. Accessed January 7, 2021.

Kayvon. My Pandemic Story: Homeless in Greater Boston for Months During Covid-19. *DigBoston.* June 24, 2020. https://digboston.com/my-pandemic-story-homeless-in-greater-boston-for-months-during-covid-19/. Accessed January 7, 2021.

Lanphear BP, Aligne CA, Auinger P, Weitzman M, Byrd RS. Residential Exposures Associated with Asthma in US Children. *Pediatrics.* 2001; 107(3) 505–511.

Mayo Clinic Staff. Lead Poisoning. Mayo Clinic website. https://www.mayoclinic.org/diseases-conditions/lead-poisoning/symptoms-causes/syc-20354717. Accessed January 7, 2021.

Mold and Dampness. American Lung Association website. https://www.lung.org/clean-air/at-home/indoor-air-pollutants/mold-and-dampness. Updated February 12, 2020. Accessed January 7, 2021.

Stein L. A Study of Respiratory Tuberculosis in Relation to Housing Conditions in Edinburgh. *British Journal of Social Medicine.* 1950; 4(3): 143–169.

Butler P. Poor Housing Linked to High Covid-19 Death Rate in London Borough. *The Guardian.* August 17, 2020. https://www.theguardian.com/world/2020/aug/17/poor-housing-linked-high-covid-19-death-rate-london-borough-brent. Accessed January 7, 2021.

Kushel MB, Gupta R, Gee L, Haas JS. Housing Instability and Food Insecurity as Barriers to Health Care Among Low-Income Americans. *Journal of General Internal Medicine.* 2006; 21(1): 71–77.

Jan T. Redlining Was Banned 50 Years Ago. It's Still Hurting Minorities Today. *The Washington Post.* March 28, 2018. https://www.washingtonpost.com/news/wonk/wp/2018/03/28/redlining-was-banned-50-years-ago-its-still-hurting-minorities-today/. Accessed January 8, 2021.

Németh J, Rowan S. Is Your Neighborhood Raising Your Coronavirus Risk? Redlining Decades Ago Set Communities Up for Greater Danger. *The Conversation.* May 26, 2020. https://theconversation.com/is-your-neighborhood-raising-your-coronavirus-risk-redlining-decades-ago-set-communities-up-for-greater-danger-138256. Accessed January 8, 2021.

Bliss L. Mapping the Lasting Effects of Redlining. *Bloomberg CityLab.* March 25, 2015. https://www.bloomberg.com/news/articles/2015-03-20/old-federal-maps-and-recent-census-data-combine-to-show-how-today-s-poverty-rates-align-with-racist-1930s-mortgaging-policies. Accessed January 8, 2021.

Rothstein R. The Racial Achievement Gap, Segregated Schools, and Segregated Neighborhoods—A Constitutional Insult. *Race and Social Problems.* 2015; 7(1): 21–30.

Hoffman JS, Shandas V, Pendleton N. The Effects of Historical Housing Policies on Resident Exposure to Intra-Urban Heat: A Study of 108 US Urban Areas. *Climate.* 2020; 8(1):12.

Rigolon A, Németh J. What Shapes Uneven Access to Urban Amenities? Thick Injustice and the Legacy of Racial Discrimination in Denver's Parks. *Journal of Planning Education and Research.* July 25, 2018.

Swanson J. Homeownership Is the Top Contributor to Household Wealth. *Mortgage News Daily.* August 28, 2019. http://www.mortgagenewsdaily.com/08282019_homeownership.asp. Accessed January 8, 2021.

Mitchell B, Franco J. HOLC "Redlining" Maps: The Persistent Structure of Segregation and Economic Inequality. National Community Reinvestment Coalition website. https://ncrc.org/holc/. Published March 20, 2018. Accessed January 8, 2021.

Leydon S. How a Long-Ago Map Created Racial Boundaries That Still Define Boston. WGBH. November 12, 2019. https://www.wgbh.org/news/local-news/2019/11/12/how-a-long-ago-map-created-racial-boundaries-that-still-define-boston. Accessed January 8, 2021.

Camire C. Map Shows How Drastically COVID-19 Risk Varies by Boston Neighborhood. American Heart Association—Eastern States website. https://easternstates.heart.org/map-shows-how-drastically-covid-19-risk-varies-by-boston-neighborhood/#:~:text=The%20map%20shows%20how%20the,than%20other%20areas%20of%20Boston.&text=The%20city%20has%20long%20struggled,its%20COVID%2D19%20risk%20spectrum. Published July 28, 2020. Accessed January 8, 2021.

MacNeill A. These 63 Massachusetts Communities Are Now in the "Red Zone" for COVID-19 Infection. Boston.com website. October 15, 2020. https://www.boston.com/news/coronavirus/2020/10/15/massachusetts-cities-towns-covid-19-red-zone-list. Accessed January 8, 2021.

Freed M, Cubanski J, Neuman T, Kates J, Michaud J. What Share of People Who Have Died of COVID-19 Are 65 and Older—and How Does It

Vary By State? Kaiser Family Foundation website. https://www.kff.org/
coronavirus-covid-19/issue-brief/what-share-of-people-who-have-
died-of-covid-19-are-65-and-older-and-how-does-it-vary-by-state/?
utm_campaign=KFF-2020-Coronavirus&utm_medium=email&_hsmi=2
&_hsenc=p2ANqtz-8ob3p-VFi8 _OMnL3f7neCnVuEOsYSu3ZRzWC9
hbZ6hExpadjvtXBz3FkZjbubTPpN1qF7d5OazNXPn68BnKbp2Pk-
4K2A&utm_ content=2&utm_source=hs_email. Published July 24, 2020.
Accessed January 8, 2021.

Mather M, Scommegna P, Kilduff L. Fact Sheet: Aging in the United States.
Population Reference Bureau website. https://www.prb.org/aging-
unitedstates-fact-sheet/. Published July 15, 2019. Accessed January 8, 2021.

Conlen M, et al. More than 100,000 US Coronavirus Deaths Are Linked
to Nursing Homes. *The New York Times*. https://www.nytimes.com/inter
active/2020/us/coronavirus-nursing-homes.html. Updated December 4,
2020. Accessed January 8, 2021.

Sinclair U, Castronovo R (Editor). *The Jungle*. New York: Oxford University
Press; 2010.

Progressive Era Investigations. US Department of Labor website. https://
www.dol.gov/general/aboutdol/history/mono-regsafepart05. Accessed
January 8, 2021.

US Bureau of Labor Statistics. News Release: National Census of Fatal
Occupational Injuries in 2018. US Bureau of Labor Statistics website.
https://www.bls.gov/news.release/archives/cfoi_12172019.pdf. Released
December 17, 2019. Accessed January 8, 2021.

Centers for Disease Control and Prevention. Achievements in Public
Health, 1900–1999 Motor-Vehicle Safety: A 20th Century Public Health
Achievement. *Morbidity and Mortality Weekly Report*. 1999; 48(18): 369–374.

The WHO European Healthy Cities Network: A Response to the COVID-19
Pandemic Close to the People. WHO Regional Office for Europe website.
https://www.euro.who.int/en/health-topics/environment-and-health/
urban-health/who-european-healthy-cities-network/the-who-european-
healthy-cities-network-a-response-to-the-covid-19-pandemic-close-to-
the-people. Accessed January 8, 2021.

Guarino B, Jacobs S. New York City, Once the US Epicenter of the
Coronavirus, Begins to Reopen. *The Washington Post*. June 8, 2020. https://
www.washingtonpost.com/nation/2020/06/08/new-york-city-once-us-
epicenter-coronavirus-begins-reopen/. Accessed January 8, 2021.

Chen DW. How Will Hudson Yards Survive the Pandemic? *The New York
Times*. June 19 2020. https://www.nytimes.com/2020/06/19/realestate/
how-will-hudson-yards-survive-the-pandemic.html. Accessed January 8,
2021.

deMause N. Pandemic Economy Could Turn a Deserted Hudson Yards
into an Even Bigger Taxpayer Money Pit. *Gothamist*. September 16, 2020.

https://gothamist.com/news/pandemic-economy-could-turn-deserted-hudson-yards-even-bigger-taxpayer-money-pit. Accessed January 8, 2021.

Kinkade S. Give Me a Lever Long Enough . . . Aspire Business Development website. https://aspirekc.com/give-me-a-lever-long-enough/. Accessed January 8, 2021.

Poe EA. The Masque of the Red Death. Project Gutenberg; 2010. https://www.gutenberg.org/files/1064/1064-h/1064-h.htm. Accessed January 8, 2021.

Chayka K. How the Coronavirus Will Reshape Architecture. *The New Yorker.* June 17, 2020. https://www.newyorker.com/culture/dept-of-design/how-the-coronavirus-will-reshape-architecture. Accessed January 8, 2021.

Wainwright O. Smart Lifts, Lonely Workers, No Towers or Tourists: Architecture After Coronavirus. *The Guardian.* April 13, 2020. https://www.theguardian.com/artanddesign/2020/apr/13/smart-lifts-lonely-workers-no-towers-architecture-after-covid-19-coronavirus. Accessed January 8, 2021.

Mann E. Story of Cities #14: London's Great Stink Heralds a Wonder of the Industrial World. *The Guardian.* April 4, 2016. https://www.theguardian.com/cities/2016/apr/04/story-cities-14-london-great-stink-river-thames-joseph-bazalgette-sewage-system. Accessed January 8, 2021.

Klein C. How Pandemics Spurred Cities to Make More Green Space for People. History website. https://www.history.com/news/cholera-pandemic-new-york-city-london-paris-green-space. Published April 27, 2020, Updated April 28, 2020. Accessed January 8, 2021.

CHAPTER 6. POLITICS, POWER, AND MONEY

Baker P, Haberman M. Trump Tests Positive for the Coronavirus. *The New York Times.* October 2, 2020. https://www.nytimes.com/2020/10/02/us/politics/trump-covid.html. Updated December 31, 2020. Accessed January 6, 2021.

Clark D. Fauci Calls Amy Coney Barrett Ceremony in Rose Garden "Superspreader Event." NBC News. October 9, 2020. https://www.nbcnews.com/politics/white-house/fauci-calls-amy-coney-barrett-ceremony-rose-garden-superspreader-event-n1242781. Accessed January 6, 2021.

Victor D, Serviss L, Paybarah A. In His Own Words, Trump on the Coronavirus and Masks. *The New York Times.* October 2, 2020. https://www.nytimes.com/2020/10/02/us/politics/donald-trump-masks.html. Accessed January 6, 2021.

Heard on Morning Edition. Trump Tells Woodward He Deliberately Downplayed Coronavirus Threat. NPR. September 10, 2020. https://www.npr.org/2020/09/10/911368698/trump-tells-woodward-he-deliberately-downplayed-coronavirus-threat. Accessed January 6, 2021.

Summers J. Timeline: How Trump Has Downplayed the Coronavirus Pandemic. NPR. October 2, 2020. https://www.npr.org/sections/latest-updates-trump-covid-19-results/2020/10/02/919432383/how-trump-has-downplayed-the-coronavirus-pandemic. Accessed January 6, 2021.

Karson K. More than Half of Americans Wear Masks as Coronavirus' New Normal Takes Hold: Poll. ABC News. April 10, 2020. https://abcnews.go.com/Politics/half-americans-wear-masks-coronavirus-normal-takes-hold/story?id=70073942. Accessed January 6, 2021.

Daily chart. In America, Even Pandemics Are Political. *The Economist*. March 11, 2020. https://www.economist.com/graphic-detail/2020/03/11/in-america-even-pandemics-are-political. Updated March 12, 2020. Accessed January 6, 2021.

Neuman S. "Maybe I'm Immune": Trump Returns to White House, Removes Mask Despite Infection. NPR. October 6, 2020. https://www.npr.org/sections/latest-updates-trump-covid-19-results/2020/10/06/920625432/maybe-i-m-immune-trump-returns-to-white-house-removes-mask-after-covid-treatment. Accessed January 6, 2021.

Alexander P. 2020. Trump Returns to White House And Removes Mask, Spurring Backlash. *Today*. October 6. https://www.youtube.com/watch?v=wyUoLqc7iL8. Accessed January 6, 2021.

The Causes of Climate Change. NASA: Climate Change and Global Warming website. https://climate.nasa.gov/causes/. Accessed January 6, 2021.

Impelli M. Fact Check: Is US "Rounding the Turn" on COVID, as Trump Claims? *Newsweek*. October 26, 2020. https://www.newsweek.com/fact-check-us-rounding-turn-covid-trump-claims-1542145. Accessed January 6, 2021.

Bryan WJ (Editor-in-Chief), Halsey FW (Associate Editor). *The World's Famous Orations*. Lincoln A. In the First Debate with Douglas. New York: Funk and Wagnalls Company; 1906. Bartleby.com website. https://www.bartleby.com/268/9/23.html. Accessed January 7, 2021.

Pigott J. The Overton Window: Some Thoughts. . . *Medium*. April 17, 2018. https://medium.com/@julianpigott/is-it-good-to-have-an-overton-window-11a6acb0884c. Accessed January 7, 2021.

Sullivan A. It Is Accomplished. *The Dish*. June 26, 2015. http://dish.andrewsullivan.com/2015/06/26/it-is-accomplished/. Accessed January 7, 2021.

Pathé S. How Democrats Came Around on Gay Rights. *Roll Call*. July 28, 2016. https://www.rollcall.com/2016/07/28/how-democrats-came-around-on-gay-rights/. Accessed January 7, 2021.

National Center for Disaster Preparedness at the Columbia University Earth Institute website. https://ncdp.columbia.edu/. Accessed January 7, 2021.

Redlener I, Sachs JD, Hansen S, Hupert N. 130,000–210,000 Avoidable COVID-19 Deaths—and Counting—in the US. Columbia University. 2020. https://ncdp.columbia.edu/custom-content/uploads/2020/10/Avoidable-COVID-19-Deaths-US-NCDP.pdf. Accessed January 7, 2021.

Earth Institute. Inadequate COVID-19 Response Likely Resulted in 130,000–210,000 Avoidable Deaths. State of the Planet website. https://blogs.ei.co lumbia.edu/2020/10/22/covid-19-response-avoidable-deaths/. Published October 22, 2020. Accessed January 7, 2021.

The Editors of the New England Journal of Medicine. Dying in a Leadership Vacuum. *The New England Journal of Medicine.* 2020; 383: 1479–1480.

Solly M. What Happened When Woodrow Wilson Came Down with the 1918 Flu? *Smithsonian Magazine.* October 2, 2020. https://www.smithsonianmag .com/smart-news/what-happened-when-woodrow-wilson-came-down-1918-flu-180975972/. Accessed January 7, 2021.

Beauchamp Z. Trump Is Mishandling Coronavirus the Way Reagan Botched the AIDS Epidemic. *Vox.* March 30, 2020. https://www.vox.com/policy-and-politics/2020/3/30/21196856/coronavirus-covid-19-trump-reagan-hiv-aids. Accessed January 7, 2021.

Rosenwald MS. "That Stain of Bloodshed": After King's Assassination, RFK Calmed an Angry Crowd with an Unforgettable Speech. *The Washington Post.* April 4, 2018. https://www.washingtonpost.com/news/retropolis/wp/2018/04/03/that-stain-of-bloodshed-after-kings-assassination-rfk-calmed-an-angry-crowd-with-an-unforgettable-speech/. Accessed January 7, 2021.

Kennedy RF. Eulogy of Martin Luther King, Jr. Indianapolis, Indiana, April 4, 1968. Speeches-USA website. http://www.speeches-usa.com/Transcripts/robert_kennedy-eulogy2.html. Accessed January 7, 2021.

Long H, Van Dam A, Fowers A, Shapiro L. The Covid-19 Recession Is the Most Unequal in Modern US History. *The Washington Post.* September 30, 2020. https://www.washingtonpost.com/graphics/2020/business/coronavirus-recession-equality/. Accessed January 7, 2021.

Laughland O. "Death by Structural Poverty": US South Struggles Against Covid-19. *The Guardian.* August 5, 2020. https://www.theguardian.com/world/2020/aug/05/us-deep-south-racism-poverty-fuel-coronavirus-pandemic. Accessed January 7, 2021.

Repairers of the Breach. Pamela Rush Memorial. https://www.youtube .com/watch?v=AT7Ka7U1DuI. Accessed January 7, 2021.

Chetty R, et al. The Association Between Income and Life Expectancy in the United States, 2001–2014. *JAMA: The Journal of the American Medical Association.* 2016; 315(16): 1750–1766.

Belluz J. What the Dip in US Life Expectancy Is Really About: Inequality. *Vox.* https://www.vox.com/science-and-health/2018/1/9/16860994/life-expectancy-us-income-inequality. Updated November 30, 2018. Accessed January 7, 2021.

Ettman CK, Cohen GH, Abdalla SM, Galea S. Do Assets Explain the Relation Between Race/Ethnicity and Probable Depression in US Adults? *PLOS One.* 2020;15(10): e0239618.

Bassett MT, Galea S. Reparations as a Public Health Priority—A Strategy for Ending Black–White Health Disparities. *The New England Journal of Medicine.* 2020; 383(22): 2101–2103.

Saavedra C. Five Ways Funders Can Support Social Movements. *Stanford Social Innovation Review.* July 9, 2018. https://ssir.org/articles/entry/five_ways_funders_can_support_social_movements. Accessed January 7, 2021.

Gerth HH (Editor), Mills CW (Editor), Weber, M. *From Max Weber: Essays in Sociology.* London: Routledge; 1991.

Opportunity Insights Economic Tracker. Track the Recovery website. https://www.tracktherecovery.org/. Accessed January 10, 2021.

CHAPTER 7. COMPASSION

Tsai J. COVID-19's Disparate Impacts Are Not a Story About Race. *Scientific American.* September 8, 2020. https://www.scientificamerican.com/article/covid-19s-disparate-impacts-are-not-a-story-about-race/. Accessed January 5, 2021.

History.com Editors. Black Death. History website. https://www.history.com/topics/middle-ages/black-death. Published September 17, 2010. Updated July 6, 2020. Accessed January 6, 2021.

The Flagellants Attempt to Repel the Black Death, 1349. EyeWitness to History website. http://www.eyewitnesstohistory.com/flagellants.htm. Accessed January 6, 2021.

The Editors of Encyclopaedia Britannica. Flagellants. Encyclopaedia Britannica website. https://www.britannica.com/topic/flagellants. Accessed January 6, 2021.

Stahl J. Herman Cain, Conservative Culture Warrior Who Opposed Mask Mandates, Dies of COVID-19. *Slate.* July 30, 2020. https://slate.com/news-and-politics/2020/07/herman-cain-mask-mandate-opponent-dies-covid-19-tulsa.html. Accessed January 6, 2021.

Reuters Staff. Herman Cain, Ex-Presidential Candidate Who Refused to Wear Mask, Dies After COVID-19 Diagnosis. Reuters. July 30, 2020. https://www.reuters.com/article/us-health-coronavirus-usa-cain/herman-cain-ex-presidential-candidate-who-refused-to-wear-mask-dies-after-covid-19-diagnosis-idUSKCN24V2OD. Accessed January 6, 2021.

Bond A. As Covid-19 Surges Among San Francisco's Homeless, Doctors Face Difficult Choices. *STAT News.* April 11, 2020. https://www.statnews.com/2020/04/11/coronavirus-san-francisco-homeless-doctors-difficult-choices/. Accessed January 6, 2021.

Berwick DM. The Moral Determinants of Health. *JAMA: The Journal of the American Medical Association.* 2020; 324(3): 225–226.

Whyte LE, Zubak-Skees C. Underlying Health Disparities Could Mean Coronavirus Hits Some Communities Harder. NPR. April 1, 2020. https://www.npr.org/sections/health-shots/2020/04/01/824874977/

underlying-health-disparities-could-mean-coronavirus-hits-some-communities-harde. Accessed January 6, 2021.

Ettman CK, Abdalla SM, Cohen GH, Sampson L, Vivier PM, Galea S. Prevalence of Depression Symptoms in US Adults Before and During the COVID-19 Pandemic. *JAMA Network Open*. 2020; 3(9): e2019686.

Couzin-Frankel J. From "Brain Fog" to Heart Damage, COVID-19's Lingering Problems Alarm Scientists. *Science*. July 31, 2020. https://www.sciencemag.org/news/2020/07/brain-fog-heart-damage-covid-19-s-lingering-problems-alarm-scientists. Accessed January 6, 2021.

Facts About Suicide. The Trevor Project website. https://www.thetrevorproject.org/resources/preventing-suicide/facts-about-suicide/. Accessed January 6, 2021.

Disparities in Breast Cancer: African American Women. American Cancer Society Cancer Action Network website. https://www.fightcancer.org/sites/default/files/FINAL%20-%20Disparities%20AABreastCancer%2002.14.17%20.pdf. Accessed January 6, 2021.

Young R, McMahon S. With Nursing Facility Closed to Visitors, This Daughter Got a Job in Laundry Room. *Here & Now*. WBUR. November 5, 2020. https://www.wbur.org/hereandnow/2020/11/05/coronavirus-nursing-home-job. Accessed January 6, 2021.

Symptoms Chart: Cold, Flu or COVID-19? *Cottage Grove Sentinel* March 16, 2020. https://cgsentinel.com/article/symptoms-chart-cold-flu-or-covid-19. Accessed January 6, 2021.

CHAPTER 8. SOCIAL, RACIAL, AND ECONOMIC JUSTICE

Seelye KQ. John Lewis, Towering Figure of Civil Rights Era, Dies at 80. *The New York Times*. July 17, 2020. https://www.nytimes.com/2020/07/17/us/john-lewis-dead.html. Updated August 4, 2020. Accessed January 5, 2021.

John Lewis: Freedom Rider. National Civil Rights Museum website. https://www.civilrightsmuseum.org/from-the-vault/posts/john-lewis-freedom-rider. Accessed January 5, 2021.

Cineas F. 6 John Lewis Speeches Key to Understanding His Work and Legacy. *Vox*. July 18, 2020. https://www.vox.com/2020/7/18/21329556/john-lewis-speeches. Accessed January 5, 2021.

Keyes A. 50 Years After March on Washington, John Lewis Still Fights. NPR. August 27, 2013. https://www.npr.org/2013/08/28/216259218/50-years-after-march-on-washington-john-lewis-still-fighting. Accessed January 5, 2021.

Stump S. Rep. John Lewis Says Martin Luther King Jr. "Would Be Very Pleased" with Protests. *Today*. June 4, 2020. https://www.today.com/news/rep-john-lewis-reflects-protests-over-george-floyd-s-death-t183286. Accessed January 5, 2021.

Adichie CN. Nigeria Is Murdering Its Citizens. *The New York Times*. October 21, 2020. https://www.nytimes.com/2020/10/21/opinion/sunday/chimamanda-adichie-nigeria-protests.html. Accessed January 5, 2021.

Nigeria: Horrific Reign of Impunity by SARS Makes Mockery of Anti-Torture Law. Amnesty International website. https://www.amnesty.org/en/latest/news/2020/06/nigeria-horrific-reign-of-impunity-by-sars-makes-mockery-of-anti-torture-law/. Published June 26, 2020. Accessed January 5, 2021.

Lawal S, Mark M. A Dozen Protesters in Nigeria Reported Killed by Security Forces. *The New York Times*. October 21, 2020. https://www.nytimes.com/2020/10/21/world/africa/nigeria-shooting-protesters-SARS-Lekki.html. Accessed January 5, 2021.

Stephens AH. Cornerstone Speech. March 21, 1861. American Battlefield Trust website. https://www.battlefields.org/learn/primary-sources/cornerstone-speech. Accessed January 5, 2021.

Cahan E. Most Home Health Aides "Can't Afford Not to Work"—Even When Lacking PPE. *Kaiser Health News*. October 16, 2020. https://khn.org/news/mostly-poor-minority-home-health-aides-lacking-ppe-share-plight-of-vulnerable-covid-patients/. Accessed January 5, 2021.

PHI. US Home Care Workers: Key Facts. 2019. PHI National website. https://phinational.org/resource/u-s-home-care-workers-key-facts-2019/. Accessed January 5, 2021.

Baer A. MLK's Efforts to Advocate Human Rights in 1967 Echoed Fifty Years Later. University of Alabama at Birmingham Institute for Human Rights website. https://sites.uab.edu/humanrights/2018/01/18/mlks-efforts-advocate-human-rights-1967-echoed-fifty-years-later/. Published January 18, 2018. Accessed January 5, 2021.

King, Jr. ML. The Three Evils of Society. An Address Delivered at the National Conference on New Politics, in Chicago, Illinois. https://www.youtube.com/watch?v=6sT9HjhocHM. Address delivered August 31, 1967. Accessed January 5, 2021.

The Veil of Ignorance. From the BBC Radio 4 series *A History of Ideas*. Scripted by Warburton N. Narrated by Fry S. Animation by Cognitive. https://www.youtube.com/watch?v=A8GDEaJtbq4. Accessed January 5, 2021.

Jefferson T. Thomas Jefferson to John Holmes, April 22, 1820. Letter. From U.S. Capitol Visitor Center Web site. https://www.visitthecapitol.gov/exhibitions/artifact/letter-thomas-jefferson-john-holmes-april-22-1820. Accessed June 22, 2021.

Miller EB. Abigail Adams. George Washington's Estate—Mount Vernon website. https://www.mountvernon.org/library/digitalhistory/digital-encyclopedia/article/abigail-adams/. Accessed January 5, 2021.

Women's Rights: Abigail Adams. US National Park Service website. https://www.nps.gov/wori/learn/historyculture/abigail-adams.htm. Updated February 26, 2015. Accessed January 5, 2021.

Asleson R. Aaron Burr: Forgotten Feminist. *Face-to-Face*. National Portrait Gallery website. https://npg.si.edu/blog/aaron-burr-forgotten-feminist. Accessed January 5, 2021.

Chase B. Coronavirus Vaccines Will Face a Deep Distrust in the Black Community. *Chicago Sun-Times*. November 20, 2020. https://chicago .suntimes.com/coronavirus/2020/11/20/21575911/coronavirus-vaccines-covid-covid19-distrust-black-community. Accessed January 5, 2021.

Nix E. Tuskegee Experiment: The Infamous Syphilis Study. History website. https://www.history.com/news/the-infamous-40-year-tuskegee-study. Published May 16, 2017. Updated December 15, 2020. Accessed January 5, 2021.

King, Jr. ML. Letter from Birmingham Jail. Martin Luther King, Jr. Research and Education Institute (Stanford University) website. http://okra.stan ford.edu/transcription/document_images/undecided/630416-019.pdf. Accessed January 5, 2021.

CHAPTER 9. HEALTH AS A PUBLIC GOOD

The Origins of Fire Fighting. Fire-Dex website. https://blog.firedex.com/ blog/2014/05/15/origins-fire-fighting. Published May 15, 2014. Accessed January 4, 2021.

Cowan D. The Richest Man in History? Crassus and Real Estate in Late Republican Rome. Macquarie University Department of Ancient History website. https://ancient-history-blog.mq.edu.au/cityOfRome/Roman-Real-Estate. Accessed January 4, 2021.

Hertzberg H. Biggus Buckus. *The New Yorker*. November 2, 2009. https:// www.newyorker.com/magazine/2009/11/09/biggus-buckus. Accessed January 4, 2021.

Galea S. Lessons from Fire Prevention: Why We Can Head Off Disease Without Sacrificing Cure. Boston University School of Public Health website. https://www.bu.edu/sph/news/articles/2017/lessons-from-fire-prevention-why-we-can-head-off-disease-without-sacrificing-cure/. Published June 11, 2017. Accessed January 4, 2021.

Haynes H. *Fire Loss in the United States During 2016*. Quincy, MA: National Fire Protection Association; Research, Data and Analytics Division; 2017.

Holmes A. Elon Musk Keeps Downplaying the Severity of Coronavirus, and Hedged His Promise to Produce Ventilators for Hospitals Mere Minutes After Making It. *Business Insider*. March 19, 2020. https://www.business insider.com/elon-musk-coronavirus-tesla-promises-experts-ventilators-controversy-2020-3. Accessed January 4, 2021.

Mitchell R. Musk Outburst over "Fascist" Coronavirus Shutdown Shows Pressure to Keep Up Growth. *Los Angeles Times*. April 30, 2020. https:// www.latimes.com/business/story/2020-04-30/tesla-musk-fremont-shutdown-outburst. Accessed January 4, 2021.

Elon Musk (@elonmusk). "Tesla is restarting production today against Alameda County rules. I will be on the line with everyone else. If anyone is arrested, I ask that it only be me."Twitter. May 11, 2020, 4:36 pm. https:// twitter.com/elonmusk/status/1259945593805221891?lang=en. Accessed January 4, 2021.

Elon Musk (@elonmusk). "FREE AMERICA NOW."Twitter. April 29, 2020, 2:14am.https://twitter.com/elonmusk/status/1255380013488189440?lang=en. Accessed January 4, 2021.

Shakespeare W. *The Life of King Henry the Fifth.* The Complete Works of William Shakespeare—MIT website. http://shakespeare.mit.edu/henryv/full.html. Accessed January 4, 2021.

Holland M. Tesla CEO Elon Musk Reports Recovery from Confirmed COVID Infection. *CleanTechnica.* November 19, 2020. https://cleantech nica.com/2020/11/19/tesla-ceo-elon-musk-reports-recovery-from-confirmed-covid-infection/. Accessed January 4, 2021.

Burki T. The Online Anti-Vaccine Movement in the Age of COVID-19. *The Lancet Digital Health.* 2020; 2(10): E504–E505.

Heilweil R. Is Social Media Ready for a Covid-19 Vaccine? *Vox.* November 9, 2020. https://www.vox.com/recode/21527013/covid-19-vaccine-pfizer-safety-social-media-misinformation. Accessed January 4, 2021.

The Learning Network. What's Going On in This Graph? | Coronavirus Protective Measures. *The New York Times.* March 26, 2020. https://www .nytimes.com/2020/03/26/learning/whats-going-on-in-this-graph-coronavirus-protective-measures.html. Accessed January 4, 2021.

Walker M, Healy J. A Motorcycle Rally in a Pandemic? "We Kind of Knew What Was Going to Happen." *The New York Times.* November 6, 2020. https://www.nytimes.com/2020/11/06/us/sturgis-coronavirus-cases.html. Accessed January 4, 2021.

Associated Press. Big Drop in Attendance Expected at Sturgis Motorcycle Rally. *Argus Leader.* August 1, 2016. https://www.argusleader.com/story/news/2016/08/01/big-drop-attendance-expected-sturgis-motorcycle-rally/87906088/. Accessed January 4, 2021.

Sturgis Motorcycle Rally 2020 website. https://www.sturgismotorcyclerally .com/. Accessed January 4, 2021.

Dave D, Friedson AI, McNichols D, Sabia JJ. The Contagion Externality of a Superspreading Event: The Sturgis Motorcycle Rally and COVID-19. IZA Discussion Paper Series. IZA—Institute of Labor Economics; 2020. http:// ftp.iza.org/dp13670.pdf. Accessed January 4, 2021.

van Wagtendonk A. As Coronavirus Cases Surge, Hospitals Are Beginning to Be Overwhelmed. *Vox.* November 21, 2020. https://www.vox.com/2020/11/21/21588959/hhs-report-coronavirus-cases-surge-hospital-staff-overwhelmed. Accessed January 4, 2021.

Hughes L, McKenney JB. What Doctors at Overwhelmed Rural Hospitals Are Facing, in Their Own Words. *Fast Company.* November 21, 2020. https://

www.fastcompany.com/90578775/what-doctors-at-overwhelmed-rural-hospitals-are-facing-in-their-own-words. Accessed January 4, 2021.

Alltucker K. "Our Neighbors, Our Family Members": Small-Town Hospitals Overwhelmed by COVID-19 Deaths. *USA Today.* November 15, 2020. https://www.usatoday.com/story/news/health/2020/11/15/hospitals-coronavirus-covid-19-cases-deaths/6267612002/. Accessed January 4, 2021.

Perrett C. The Outbreak in North Dakota Is So Bad That Healthcare Workers Can Now Keep Treating COVID-19 Patients Even if They Have the Disease. *Business Insider.* November 10, 2020. https://www.businessinsider.com/north-dakota-nurses-keep-working-covid-19-2020-11. Accessed January 4, 2021.

The Constitution of the United States. Preamble. United States Senate website. https://www.senate.gov/civics/constitution_item/constitution.htm. Accessed January 4, 2021.

CHAPTER 10. UNDERSTANDING WHAT MATTERS MOST

Belluz J. Who Will Get the Covid-19 Vaccine First? A CDC Advisory Panel Just Weighed In. *Vox.* December 2, 2020. https://www.vox.com/2020/12/2/21754854/covid-19-vaccine-cdc-advisory-recommendation. Accessed January 4, 2021.

History.com Editors. French Revolution. History website. https://www.history.com/topics/france/french-revolution. Published November 9, 2009. Updated October 26, 2020. Accessed January 4, 2021.

Laborie S. Work: The Raft of the Medusa. The Louvre website. https://www.louvre.fr/en/oeuvre-notices/raft-medusa. Accessed January 4, 2021.

Géricault T. *The Raft of the Medusa.* 1819. The Louvre Museum. Paris, France. Copied from Wikimedia Commons website. https://commons.wikimedia.org/wiki/File:JEAN_LOUIS_THÉODORE_GÉRICAULT_-_La_Balsa_de_la_Medusa_(Museo_del_Louvre,_1818-19).jpg. Accessed January 4, 2021.

Peregrine A. Raft of the Medusa: A Grisly Tale of Incompetence and Cannibalism. *The Telegraph.* July 12, 2016. https://www.telegraph.co.uk/travel/destinations/europe/france/articles/raft-of-the-medusa-louvre-explained/. Accessed January 4, 2021.

Andone D, Moshtaghian A. A Person Who Was Covid-19 Positive Attended a Church Service and Exposed 180 People, Officials Say. CNN. May 17, 2020. https://www.cnn.com/2020/05/17/us/covid-19-mothers-day-church-exposure/index.html. Accessed January 4, 2021.

Hummer RA, Hernandez EM. The Effect of Educational Attainment on Adult Mortality in the US. Population Reference Bureau website. https://www.prb.org/us-educational-attainment-mortality/. Published July 18, 2013. Accessed January 4, 2021.

Vulnerable Populations: Education Level. University of California San Francisco Smoking Cessation Leadership Center website. https://smokingcessationleadership.ucsf.edu/education-level. Accessed January 4, 2021.

Galea S. A Good Education—the Best Prevention? Boston University School of Public Health website. https://www.bu.edu/sph/news/articles/2016/a-good-education-the-best-prevention/. Published May 8, 2016. Accessed January 4, 2021.

Kamenetz A. Are the Risks of Reopening Schools Exaggerated? NPR. October 21, 2020. https://www.npr.org/2020/10/21/925794511/were-the-risks-of-reopening-schools-exaggerated. Accessed January 4, 2021.

Greenwood M. Still Wiping Down Your Grocery Store Purchases? Coronavirus Risk Is "Exceedingly Small," Experts Say. *USA Today*. September 8, 2020. https://www.usatoday.com/story/news/nation/2020/09/08/do-you-still-need-wipe-down-grocery-store-takeout-boxes/5743240002/. Accessed January 4, 2021.

Colarossi N. Watch: Crying CA Restaurant Owner Says She's Losing "Everything" While Mayor Allows Neighboring Movie Set to Stay Open. *Newsweek*. December 5, 2020. https://www.newsweek.com/watch-crying-ca-restaurant-owner-says-shes-losing-everything-while-mayor-allows-neighboring-1552607. Accessed January 4, 2021.

Bavli I, Sutton B, Galea S. Harms of Public Health Interventions Against Covid-19 Must Not Be Ignored. *BMJ*. 2020; 371: m4074.

Pattani A. Amid COVID and Racial Unrest, Black Churches Put Faith in Mental Health Care. *Kaiser Health News*. December 1, 2020. https://khn.org/news/amid-covid-and-racial-unrest-black-churches-put-faith-in-mental-health-care/. Accessed January 4, 2021.

Watts J. Did Mother's Day Church Services Help Spread Coronavirus In Northern California? CBS Sacramento website. https://sacramento.cbslocal.com/2020/05/25/mothers-day-covid19-outbreak/. Published May 25, 2020. Accessed April 26, 2021.

CHAPTER 11. WORKING IN COMPLEXITY AND DOUBT

Raache H. COVID-19 Surges Once Again in Oklahoma with 35 More Deaths, over 3,900 New Cases. KFOR-TV website. https://kfor.com/news/coronavirus/covid-19-surges-once-again-in-oklahoma-with-35-more-deaths-over-3900-new-cases/. Published December 12, 2020. Accessed January 3, 2021.

McFarling UL. "They've Been Following the Science": How the Covid-19 Pandemic Has Been Curtailed in Cherokee Nation. *STAT News*. November 17, 2020. https://www.statnews.com/2020/11/17/how-covid19-has-been-curtailed-in-cherokee-nation/. Accessed January 3, 2021.

Hatcher SM, et al. COVID-19 Among American Indian and Alaska Native Persons—23 States, January 31–July 3, 2020. *Morbidity and Mortality Weekly Report.* 2020; 69(34): 1166–1169.

Miller K. Oklahoma Governor: No Mandate Masks Despite Recommendation. Associated Press. September 17, 2020. https://apnews.com/article/virus-outbreak-oklahoma-oklahoma-city-210cc5dfbdceob65a1a1b7991c3f3b04. Accessed January 3, 2021.

The Black Death. National Archives (UK) website. https://www.nationalar chives.gov.uk/museum/item.asp?item_id=23. Accessed January 3, 2021.

Wilson KM, Brady TJ, Lesesne C, on behalf of the NCCDPHP Work Group on Translation. An Organizing Framework for Translation in Public Health: The Knowledge to Action Framework. *Preventing Chronic Disease.* 2011; 8(2): A46.

Hempel J. Social Media Made the Arab Spring, but Couldn't Save It. *Wired.* January 26, 2016. https://www.wired.com/2016/01/social-media-made-the-arab-spring-but-couldnt-save-it/. Accessed January 3, 2021.

Ruston S. John Keats, Poet-Physician. British Library website. https://www.bl.uk/romantics-and-victorians/articles/john-keats-poet-physician. Published May 15, 2014. Accessed January 4, 2021.

Keats J, Gittings R (Editor), revised by Mee J. *John Keats: Selected Letters.* New York: Oxford University Press; 2002.

Sacerdote B, Sehgal R, Cook M. Why Is All COVID-19 News Bad News? National Bureau of Economic Research working paper no. w28110. https://www.nber.org/papers/w28110. Accessed January 4, 2021.

Roberts S. Flattening the Coronavirus Curve. *The New York Times.* March 27, 2020. https://www.nytimes.com/article/flatten-curve-coronavirus.html. Accessed January 4, 2021.

The Coronavirus Has Pushed 3.3m American Workers onto the Dole in a Week. *The Economist.* March 26, 2020. https://www.economist.com/graphic-detail/2020/03/26/the-coronavirus-has-pushed-33m-american-workers-onto-the-dole-in-a-week. Accessed January 4, 2021.

Chernow R. *Grant.* New York: Penguin Press; 2017.

Welna D. Coronavirus Has Now Killed More Americans than Vietnam War. NPR. April 28, 2020. https://www.npr.org/sections/coronavirus-live-updates/2020/04/28/846701304/pandemic-death-toll-in-u-s-now-exceeds-vietnam-wars-u-s-fatalities. Accessed January 4, 2021.

Goldberg C, Mitchell K (guest contributor). Remembrance: Public Health Lessons From the Janitor and the Melon Lady. *CommonHealth.* WBUR. June 7, 2012. https://www.wbur.org/commonhealth/2012/06/07/public-health-bill-bicknell. Accessed January 4, 2021.

El-Sayed AM, Galea S (Editors). *Systems Science and Population Health.* New York: Oxford University Press; 2017.

Keyes K, Galea S. What Matters Most: Quantifying an Epidemiology of Consequence. *Annals of Epidemiology.* 2015; 25(5): 305–311.

CHAPTER 12. HUMILITY AND INFORMING THE PUBLIC CONVERSATION

McFarling UL. A "Duty to Warn": An ER Doctor, Shaped by War and Hardship, Chronicles the Searing Realities of Covid-19. *STAT News.* December 21, 2020. https://www.statnews.com/2020/12/21/duty-to-warn-doctor-shaped-by-war-hardship-chronicles-searing-realities-of-covid19/. Accessed January 3, 2021.

Sargent L. On Epistemic Humility and Privilege. Moral Guillotines website. https://moralguillotines.wordpress.com/2019/04/23/on-epistemic-humility-and-privilege/. Published April 23, 2019. Accessed January 3, 2021.

Bonea P. 8 Profound Meanings to "I Know That I Know Nothing." Hasty Reader website. https://hastyreader.com/the-only-thing-i-know-is-that-i-know-nothing/. Accessed January 3, 2021.

Space.com Staff. Private Space Pioneer Elon Musk Counters Neil Armstrong, Critics on "60 Minutes." Space.com website. https://www.space.com/14936-spacex-ceo-elon-musk-60-minutes-interview.html. Published March 16, 2012. Accessed January 3, 2021.

Mars & Beyond. SpaceX website. https://www.spacex.com/human-spaceflight/mars/. Accessed January 3, 2021.

Sheffield R. Bob Dylan Has Given Us One of His Most Timely Albums Ever with "Rough and Rowdy Ways." *Rolling Stone.* June 15, 2020. https://www.rollingstone.com/music/music-album-reviews/bob-dylan-rough-rowdy-ways-1015086/. Accessed January 3, 2021.

The Nobel Prize in Literature 2016. The Nobel Prize website. https://www.nobelprize.org/prizes/literature/2016/summary/. Accessed January 3, 2021.

Dylan B. Bob Dylan Nobel Lecture. Nobel Prize website. https://www.nobelprize.org/prizes/literature/2016/dylan/lecture/. Accessed January 3, 2021.

Wolfson E, Wilson C. Tracking the Spread of the Coronavirus Outbreak Around the US and the World. *Time.* March 11, 2020. https://time.com/5800901/coronavirus-map/. Updated January 3, 2021. Accessed January 3, 2021.

Charles S. Pamela Rush Exposed the Injustice of Poverty in Rural Alabama . Ultimately It Stole Her Life. *Montgomery Advertiser.* July 12, 2020. https://www.montgomeryadvertiser.com/story/news/2020/07/12/pamela-rush-exposed-poverty-sewage-waste-water-rural-al-died-coronavirus/5408146002/. Accessed January 3, 2021.

Roberts M, Reither EN, Lim S. Contributors to the Black–White Life Expectancy Gap in Washington D.C. *Scientific Reports.* 2020; 10: 13416.

Galea S. The Real Reason Why American Lives Are Getting Shorter. *HuffPost.* December 7, 2018. https://www.huffpost.com/entry/opinion-life-expectancy-americans_n_5c0982b0e4b0b6cdaf5d37c8. Accessed January 3, 2021.

Goodnough A, Hoffman J. The Elderly vs. Essential Workers: Who Should Get the Coronavirus Vaccine First? *The New York Times.* December 5, 2020.

https://www.nytimes.com/2020/12/05/health/covid-vaccine-first.html.
Updated December 20, 2020. Accessed January 3, 2021.
Sullivan A. Why 2021 Is Going to Be Epic. *The Weekly Dish*. December 18,
2020. https://andrewsullivan.substack.com/p/why-2021-is-going-to-be-
epic. Accessed January 3, 2021.
Milton J, Leonard J (Editor). *Paradise Lost*. London: Penguin Classics; 2000.
Pollack-Pelzner D. Shakespeare Wrote His Best Works During a Plague. *The
Atlantic*. March 14, 2020. https://www.theatlantic.com/culture/archive/
2020/03/broadway-shutdown-could-be-good-theater-coronavirus/
607993/. Accessed January 3, 2021.

EPILOGUE

Kennedy RF. Eulogy of Martin Luther King, Jr. Indianapolis, Indiana, April 4,
1968. Speeches-USA website. http://www.speeches-usa.com/Transcripts/
robert_kennedy-eulogy2.html. Accessed January 1, 2021.
Baldwin J. *The Fire Next Time*. New York: Vintage Books; (1963) 1993.
The Fire Next Time by James Baldwin. The British Library website. https://
www.bl.uk/collection-items/the-fire-next-time-by-james-baldwin.
Accessed January 1, 2021.

Index

Page numbers followed by *f* refer to figures.